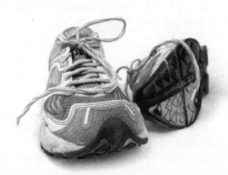

Faith & Fitness

Diet and Exercise for a Better World

Revised and Updated

ISBN-978-0-615-69364-4
Manufactured in the USA
By :Worzalla Publishing Co., Stevens Point, WI

Original edition, 2007
"Faith & Fitness: Diet and Exercise for a Better World"
Augsburg Fortress, Publishers,
Box 1209, Minneapolis, MN 55440-1209.
ISBN-13:978-0-8066-5331-0
Rights of Original Publication, repurchased by author, 2011.

Acclaim for *Faith and Fitness:*

"Faith and Fitness contains within its pages sound theological foundation for holistic health."
(Circuit Rider) The United Methodist Church

"This book is for all Christians who have a deep concern for social justice, advocates better self-care for the purpose of caring for others and the planet"
Publisher's weekly

"An abundance of wisdom and helpful advice on the topics of nutrition and exercise."
The Catholic Review

"Filled with practical ideas about food, exercise, and total wellness, the book explores the connections between real and spiritual sustenance, affluence, and exercise and the relationship between a healthy congregation and healthy individuals."
Evangelical Lutheran Church in America (Seeds for the Parish)

"This hippie-preacher who is more U2's Bono than Billy Graham says the real focus should be consuming the right amount of food ourselves and saving the excess resources for the millions dying of hunger."
USA Today

"Rev. Hafer offers weight-loss salvation through God."
E! Entertainment Television

"'Faith and Fitness' literally changed my life!"
Chaplain, Hickman Air Force Base

"For someone like me whose life motto is "faith, family, fitness," this book is a must-read. Besides all his very useful tips about proper diet and necessary exercise, Hafer scores big as he powerfully describes how-as we maintain the vigorous activities our bodies are designed for-we are not only enhancing our lives, but are better equipped to serve others, goals every one of us should want to achieve."
Les Steckel, former NFL coach &
President, Fellowship of Christian Athletes, Kansas, MO

Put your motives and preconceptions aside and prepare to have a different journey that helps you forge a new and clearer understanding of faith and fitness…in an era of affluence. Tom's book takes readers to the Bible basics when it comes to food and exercise. Tom's message couldn't be more clear; eat authentic food and move your body…That is God's designed prescription for healthy living…Without this prescriptive, exercise has little value. With it, God breathes life into your physical pursuits.
Brad Bloom, publisher of Faith & Fitness Magazine

This soul searching message challenges each one of us to pursue a more inspirational life to take care of the environment, our health, and to bring about the ultimate of caring for each other and world peace. This book touches our hearts.
Ardath Rodale, chairman of the board of Rodale Inc.

"Faith and Fitness puts into perspective that being healthy and fit is more than exercise and nutrition. You need to be spiritually fit as well. This book creates an awareness of the daily requirements we need to be healthy physically and spiritually. The book has inspiration with perspiration!"
Lance Shore, Vice President Torque Fitness

"Faith and Fitness demonstrates three changes that can result in faithful and happy lives. First is a shift away from money toward love as the primary motivator for our actions. Second is the move away from a need to lose weight model towards one focused on the need to feed others. Third is the shift to honor our bodies so as to care for others. Packed with practical information and advice about eating and exercising, this down-to-earth book helps us move toward compassionate faith. Hafer's claim is that it will also make us both spiritually and physically more healthy!"

Shannon Jung, professor at Saint Paul School of Theology, Kansas City Author of Sharing Food and Food for Life (Fortress Press).

"Tom Hafer's understanding of the spiritual responsibility we have toward care for the land is clearly in line with...Biblical teachings as caretakers (not exploiters) of the earth...Faith and Fitness outlines the link between caring for the land and the effects the food will have on our bodies."

Stan Doerr, Executive Director
Educational Concerns for Hunger Organization (ECHO)

"The best motivation for doing anything is love. Lasting motivation for fitness does not come from the temporary self satisfaction of looking good to ourselves in the mirror and/or to others at class reunions or other events. Lasting motivation for exercise comes from love. Love of the Lord and the marvelous body He created for us. Love of family, friends and the ability to serve and care for them. Love of the knowledge that we are doing the right thing for ourselves and others. Tom's great suggestions for diet and exercise are but a part of a larger vision for a world made better through the lasting motivation of love."

5 out of 5 stars The Best Motivation, "A Kid's Review"
(Amazon April 16, 2010)

Contents

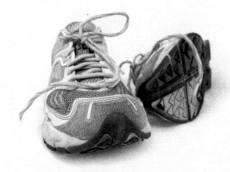

Faith & Fitness

To view the inner workings of that rarely-seen world that is inside the human body, the medical student can only stand and marvel as he learns; that is, if he does not miss the forest as he studies the trees. It has become my deepest passion to teach others to care for the greatest tool for which they have been gifted—their own body. It is the one body that they are entrusted to be a good steward of during their lifetime. With care, it will be animated for a hopeful one-hundred years and then returned to the elements in which it came...

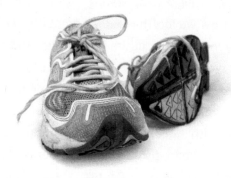

Introduction

Since the release of the first manuscript in 2006, *Faith & Fitness* and the accompanied workshops have found homes in a large diversity of locations. Interestingly, a myriad of people and congregations who might not always agree on areas of theology, have found unity when it comes to the importance of our health and wellness. That spiritual unity is rooted in the understanding that we are truly called to care for ourselves so that we can better care for others. This understanding has been the motivation that can last us throughout our years far more effectively than the motivation of weight-loss for "aesthetic" reasons. It should be no surprise to readers that aesthetics or how we *look* is largely how weight-loss, eating right, and exercise is marketed. How we *look* has a deep emotional connection to most everyone. It is our desire to look slim and healthy, not fat. When we care for ourselves to better care for others, our deep emotional quest for fitness goes deeper still.

Over the years, I have had the honor to speak and correspond with hundreds of congregations, pastors, and priests of the Methodist, Catholic, Lutheran, Presbyterian, Assemblies of God, Baptist, Episcopalian, Non-Denominational, Evangelical, United Church of Christ, Reformed, Pentecostal, Jehovah's Witness Kingdom Halls, and Mennonite churches. I also had the privilege to speak to faith-based organizations like *Volunteers of America* as well as a host of secular and business communities. Also, the *Faith & Fitness* concept had found its way into many civic, social, and military organizations like Rotary, Kiwanis, Veteran's of Foreign Wars, and others.

To some degree, it seems like everyone is interested in the topic of fitness. "Caring for ourselves to better care for others" has fueled a motivation that *preaches* across denominations, non-religions, and even folks outside the Christian circle. Yes, interestingly enough, *Faith & Fitness* has also allowed some wonderful fruitful inter-faith dialogue with Buddhists, Hindus, Muslims, Jewish Congregations, and individuals. It seems that personal health is a universal desire.

I have also found that there is potential to speak the same language in faith to an academic arena that often times shuns the religious, but now is finding a budding interest in the connection between faith and wellbeing.

You will find that this revised and updated edition of *Faith & Fitness* has a wider reach than the original. In other words, the emphasis is on the common goodwill that binds us all together. A unity of our common faith is often referred to as "Ecumenism" (Ecumenism, can be loosely interpreted from its Greek root as meaning "the whole inhabited world").

As Christians, when reaching outside our usual and comfortable Christian circles, we have a greater opportunity to reach lives with hope as Jesus did. It is the *Mother Teresa Effect* in spreading good news. Her effectiveness in spreading God's hope was not in her talking of God. Her talk was more effective through her *service* to the world. She 'walked the talk', so to speak. She embodied the hands of Jesus to the Hindu orphans of Calcutta. She was love in work clothes. Her actions told God's love story far more effectively than words could.

When we take time to reach out to spread health and wellness to all of God's people with our efforts, regardless of creeds or religions, we have the potential to be the embodied caring hands of Christ without the need of words. Words more often do not reach the depth of caring that a single act of kindness can. Helping someone get healthy is a single profound caring act. Through our actions, we walk the talk of the religion we are professing.

I think you will find this edition will attempt to do just that. Even though it is updated with the latest in research, the core "take home" is the same. It boils down to three principles. Those principles are the following:

1. **Food:** *Everything we need for sustaining health and wellness has been provided for us through nature since the beginning. If not true, life would not be. Today's health crisis is not the fault of the individual, but is a manifestation of our community forgetting our blessings of real, whole, natural foods, and simple life-giving fresh water.*

2. **Exercise:** *Unlike anything we create by hand, like a car or a refrigerator which starts to breakdown when used, the body improves in every way with moderate to heavy use. Exercise is a magic pill, a fountain of youth, an anti-depressant. The body is improved in every way possible, naturally with exercise. The Creator intended for us to move and move a lot for optimum health by design.*

3.   **Faith:** *Our efforts made towards personal fitness can become a true spiritual discipline, an expression of gratitude and thanksgiving for all of life. When we 'care for ourselves to better care for others', we simplify and intensify our quest towards personal fitness.*

Faith & Fitness is not attempting to be religious. It is an attempt to explore the health and wellness for humankind as seen through the eyes of our Divine Creator. With that understanding, we can discover what our Creator intended for us to do to be healthy and well, reasonably and naturally, without the confines of fad diets, trendy exercise gadgets and programs, or even confining religious dogma or doctrine.

For humanity to flourish, we are obligated to share the goodness of God's provisions with **all** people. Likewise, **all** religions teach us to 'love one another'. Love is best demonstrated through simple acts of compassionate service. We are called to practice "The Golden Rule": Do unto others as you would have them do unto you. This is not only a Christian doctrine. It is the center of all religions.

Islam, Judaism, Buddhism, and Hinduism all echo this understanding with Christians: we are to care for our neighbors, especially those neighbors who are poor, sick, frail, elderly, disabled, and any others who cannot care for themselves.

The Qur'an, the Muslim Holy Scripture, says the following: *Righteousness is this: that one should give away wealth out of love for him to the near of kin and the orphans and the needy and the wayfarer and the beggars and for the emancipation of the captives. Those are the ones who have been true, and it is those who are the righteous (2.177).* The Old Testament prophets warn early Jews against neglecting the orphans, the poor, and the forgotten. Buddha said, *"If you do not tend to one another, then who is there to tend to you? Whoever would tend me, he should tend the sick" (Vinaya, Mahavagga 8:26.3).* And of course Jesus' mandate to love one another is found throughout all the New Testament scriptures. We are called to be our brother's keeper. The ancient Talmud asks us *"if not you, then who?"*

By embracing our brothers and sisters in community through love, all things are possible. Wars end, hungry mouths are fed, health improves, opportunity knocks, populations stabilize, the earth restores its resources, and a deeper revelation of God's love exists for everyone regardless of their doctrine.

So, our new motivation towards health practices reflects 'doing unto others as you would have them do unto you'.

When we care for ourselves to better care for others, we are practicing *The Golden Rule.*

We have the perspective of seeing each other in the image of God, completely 'inter-dependent' on the goodwill of each other, by design. This is reason enough to celebrate the things that are best for all of us. We celebrate together proper diet and purposeful exercise. We give thanks for our health.

I learned to truly celebrate life by sitting at the feet of the thousands of older adults that I have had the opportunity to work with both in physical therapy and as a chaplain. I often think of just how lucky I was to be put in such a unique position. My career path wasn't of my choosing. But looking back, I realize that I was exactly where I needed to be.

At twenty-two years old, I started a physical therapy clinic after college that started to do fairly well, financially. It was to be a sports medicine clinic in southern Florida. Its purpose was to care for high school, collegiate, and community athletes; as well as, high-profile professional athletes with vacation homes in the area. That was my hope. What I ended up with was a large clinic full of senior citizens whose goals and abilities had nothing to do with athletics. Instead, they were concerned with functional activities, such as strengthening their legs to get out of a chair or walking up stairs. Those were the people with whom I worked. It wasn't the NBA or the NFL, but simply senior citizens who wished to learn to walk again. I didn't intend it that way, it was just the way the next two decades panned out.

After physical therapy school, I had even taken an additional two years to receive my Athletic Training Certification in order to become more marketable in the community as a sports medicine provider. In the early years, I would ask myself, "why did I spend all those years in college for sports medicine when I am working with the elderly?"

Although it wasn't my design, the work became fairly lucrative. Services for seniors were in high demand, and they paid accordingly. So, while some of my former sports medicine classmates were in exciting careers with universities and assisting a few professional sports teams; I was working hard with seniors in my little corner of the Sunshine State.

Like most young Americans fresh out of college, I followed the dream of working and earning my fortune. I worked hard. Despite the success, something was missing. My diet was poor. My once disciplined exercise routine was now sporadic. Imagine—a guy who studied nothing but sports medicine, exercise, and nutrition was neither exercising nor eating well! I had (and still have) a wonderful wife, three incredible children, a large home, and that successful business. But, at that point, my spiritual life was feeble; out of balance.

I have the senior citizens to thank for my early success. After all, they trusted in me, which is why they came for physical therapy. But I was entrusted with something more than their hope to restore their weakened bodies. In addition to receiving medical services, they told me their stories.

It was the stories they shared that eventually made the real impact. Out of all age groups, the elderly take the time to communicate through stories most often. Initially, I took the stories they shared with me at face value. There was variety in the joys and sorrows, regrets and accomplishments they shared, but one lesson to learn was clear. It was the common thread present in some form in every account. Stories of thousands of older adults told me again and again what I, an ambitious young person, needed to hear. That lesson was loud and clear. That lesson was: *"don't be a fool"*.

Out of love and concern, my patients were warning me to find my balance; to treasure what I have that matters most; and not be a fool. *"For where your treasure is, there your heart will be also" (Luke 12:34).*

There are moments when God speaks. Oftentimes, the voice is so subtle that we choose to ignore it. If we listen, truly listen, it is usually such a profound revelation that the very pattern of our lives is shaken and the foundation shifts. Such a revelation came to me on December 15, 1997.

I had just sold my first physical therapy clinic. I turned a profit and quickly started my plans to do it all over again. I faced long and late hours. It was then that my four-year-old son, Daniel, received a five-dollar bill in the mail for his birthday from his great-grandmother. As I was leaving for work that morning, I noticed Daniel holding his crisp bill tightly. At that time, my wife was the one who kept things organized and made sure the needs of our three young children were met. I didn't have time for such things—after all, I was the successful breadwinner. But that morning I decided to make a promise to Daniel: "I will come home early and take you to the store to spend your five dollars".

As I left, I couldn't help but wonder what he would decide to get. After all, five dollars is big money for a preschooler, especially at the time. He loved candy and could get a lot of it for that. But maybe he would want a water pistol.

Throughout the day, I continued to wonder what Daniel's mystery purchase would be. I was proud of my plan to take valuable time out of my important business schedule to drive him to the store to spend his gift money.

At 5:30 P.M., I walked into my home and was greeted by my preschool son descending the stairs, smiling slightly, and trying hard to contain his enthusiasm. With his hand outstretched and clutching the five-dollar bill, Daniel said, "Here, you take this money, Daddy. Then you won't have to work so much".

Soon after that, we sold the big house, took our first real family vacation, started eating healthy, and exercised regularly. I began working only forty hours a week. Within a few years, we relocated our family to a more modest inexpensive home out of the city. The reduction in the mortgage allowed me to attend seminary. The goal was to gain a deeper understanding of God's hope for me. The goal was to never to be disillusioned again.

What is God calling you to? What a horrible tragedy—to reach the end of life discovering that accomplishments one pursued were left wanting. I learned this lesson in time, and my hope is that you will learn it too. Think of this as a financial self-help book with a goal of exposing the shortcomings of material pursuits to the exclusion of healthy self-fulfillment. While it is obviously a book about fitness—emphasizing disability-free living through diet and exercise—another goal of this book is to help you realize the deeper value of the people placed carefully in your life.

But, most importantly, I hope you find this to be a book that offers the complementary balance between fitness and the faith you profess. I realize that these hopes are tall orders for one thin publication. But you will see that through dynamic 'paradigm shifts' (or changes of thinking), fitness will find its proper place for you personally which will deliberately effect your community of family and friends for the better. You will even contribute in some small way to global-healing spiritually, physically, and environmentally.

I warn you that this publication will not teach you the steps to be rich. You will not learn tricks for quick weight loss; and it won't help you find a better career, get a bigger house, or look younger (there are plenty of books that claim they can help you with those things). Rather, this book should convince you that the rabbit trails we chase to improve our looks, our wealth, and our position all fail to provide us with the fulfilling life we receive as a proponent of *The Golden Rule*. Together, we can respond to God's call to be good stewards of our own health, our neighbors' health, and the health of our planet. May the stories you tell as a senior to younger generations be joyful, colorful, and of good health!

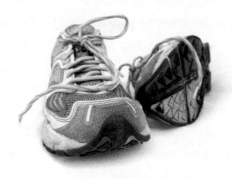

Food

Everything we need for sustaining health and wellness has been provided for us through nature since the beginning. If not true, life would not be. Today's health crisis is not the fault of the individual, but is a manifestation of our community forgetting our blessings of real, whole, natural foods, and simple life-giving fresh water.

Like millions of older adults who grew up as children of the Great Depression, Alice remembers the struggles her parents went through in order to provide food for her brothers and sisters. She would say, "You just did what you had to do, there was not a choice, no handouts, and everyone scrambled to support each other". Hunger was a painful truth. Now in her nineties, Alice and millions of her contemporaries, could not imagine wasting food. She couldn't consider taking more than her share knowing someone else might be in need.

An interesting change has taken place in the food industry since World War II. From the humble beginnings of simple agriculture—before fortifying and enriching, mass farming, pesticides, insecticides, commercial canning, frozen and fast foods—the food industry has evolved into the ubiquitous giant it is today.

Over the years, the food we eat has changed drastically. Food is now globally prepackaged and processed. Whereas, for the six to ten thousand years prior to modern times; it was eaten directly after harvesting, whole and raw. As early as 1939, it was said that Mother Nature "included all the necessary vitamins in basic raw food materials" and "modern food processing and preserving methods impaired the potency of these vitamins"; but people continued to buy processed foods with additives instead of fresh foods. It was also understood early that those advocating food *fads*, like new diet products, were more successful in gaining acceptance for their ideas than were the 'tried and true' professional nutritionists. As early as 1959, Time Magazine stated: "the emphasis in the food business has moved more and more from manufacturing to marketing".

As early as 2002 - if we include all aspects from the farm and fertilizer to the restaurant and dinner table - the food industry reached 13 percent of the Gross National Product, passing a trillion dollars. It has only risen higher in the last 10 years. In America, we produce enough food to give approximately 3,800 calories daily to each American. This is nearly twice the amount that is required or recommended by the United States Department of Agriculture (USDA) for individuals. Food is evolving cheaper per calorie and there is exponentially more calories available per American.

A startling and paradoxical truth that we face is that we spend considerably more and more each year on marketed diets, obesity solutions, and related surgeries ($60 billion in 2010); yet, the obesity rate and related chronic illnesses among Americans continues to rise each year.

We have a surplus of food within our grasp. Food companies all compete for our attention by making their products more appealing to our tastes; as well as, making sure food is as convenient as it can be for overconsumption. Meanwhile, more than a billion people worldwide don't know where their next meal will come from.

Our more than a trillion dollar food industry tells us to "eat more". Our doctors say "eat less". We wish we could control ourselves and not eat so much; especially, while so many go without food. Our *'gut'* tells us that something is fundamentally flawed with our current food surplus scenario. This *gut* feeling is truly the start of our awakening to redirecting the momentum of this great imbalance.

> *"We search for more answers because the ones we have found are not to our liking."*
> —Joel Fuhrman, M.D. Eat to Live

The diet industry continues to strive for new products and new weight loss "cures". As early as 1960, $500 million was spent on food fads, extreme diets, and cure-alls (obesity surgeries were not invented yet). As mentioned before, that number has risen to $60 billion in 2010. This is a 1200% increase in the 50 years between 1960 and 2010 on spending for hopeful weight loss miracles.

Because weight loss is an emotional and sometimes desperate issue; the products sell even if they are not thoroughly researched and deemed as safe. Many times, if a "cure" for weight loss is advertised, it will be purchased by the hopeful user even if found unsafe. A weight-loss product in the 1990s was a top seller even though it was linked to eight hundred side effects and at least twenty deaths. In spite of those warnings, the sales were still steady in the millions. Unfortunately, this was not a one-time case. Weight-loss products continue to sell, whatever warnings they carry. New products in different forms and packages are all advertised to be the shortcut solution to wellness and permanent *slimness*. The nation continues to pay billions on false hope.

We fight having an abundance of food; while outside our land of excess milk and honey, our neighbors starve. Starvation and obesity are food distribution problems.

If that *gut* feeling were to spark the conscience of millions of Americans, then a shift would happen from the current "need-to-lose-weight" belief or paradigm to a "need-to-feed-others" paradigm. If this were to happen, then this nation would lose weight and get healthy more easily. More importantly, we would feed the hungry. Ultimately, this shift in our thinking motivates us not to focus on our own weight or health problems; but on the needs of our global community. By broadening our mission from our personal weight issues to the health of the global community, we demonstrate compassionate wellness; and our personal weight and health issues become significantly less challenging. The switch from struggling with our own abundance to addressing the needs of our neighbors will awaken our deeper *hunger* that is not satisfied with food: the instinctive need to practice *The Golden Rule.*

That which is true, right, or good awakens in us a deeper understanding of purpose. Acting on behalf of our neighbors in the Third World or at home is a major step toward this monumental shift of thinking. When someone with abundance is emotionally and spiritually connected to the billion with no food; he or she becomes acutely aware of the injustice of the imbalance of food distribution in the world. Without the experience of seeing it firsthand, one's biggest food decisions might include deciding which restaurant to go to or whether to eat a second or third helping at the all-you-can-eat buffet! With a paradigm shift, the appetite for *excess* is lost. Overeating causes guilt, not only because one might gain weight, but because of the deep compassion for those who have nothing. It is hard to overeat when remembering the face of a child who goes without food, a child whose only crime is to be born in an unfortunate impoverished place.

We have been very well trained on food do's and don'ts. But focusing on food control still keeps one's mind on food and not on the bigger picture. When we think with deeper compassion for the poor, we take a bold step back to refocus. Eating only our share of healthier and more natural foods, we could feed the poor with our abundance. We would "feed" a healthy and moral way of thinking.

Rabbi Harold Kushner tells of a Native American Indian tribal leader who describes his daily struggle of right and wrong as two dogs that fight for position. One dog is right (truth, good) and the other is wrong (untruth, bad). When a listener asks which dog usually wins, he responds, "The one I feed the most". Feed what is good and right to feed.

Self-awareness through occasional fasting also creates the deeper understanding of those who go without. Hunger pangs remind us vividly and concretely of those who have nothing. Fasting enhances our appreciation of the food we do have as well. The individual can end a fast by simply going to the cupboard or refrigerator. Those who are impoverished do not have that luxury. The prayers of fasting individuals are deeper and more appreciative of the food they are about to receive. After fasting, one treats food differently, with a new respect. Never again will one complain about food overabundance with a full mouth once they felt the 'pangs' of true hunger. Never again will one feel that food overabundance is a curse.

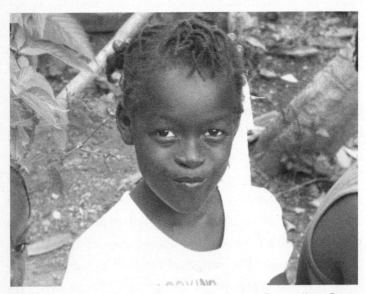

One of many memorable young faces outside Port-au-Prince, Haiti. Picture taken by author six weeks following January 2010 earthquake. The child *and* the mission party were healthier and better nourished because they shared the dinner table.

Real Food

An intriguing twenty-five-year study of the longest-living people in the world suggests that diet, exercise, faith practices, and personal relationships are the reasons for their longevity. The people of Okinawa, located off the coast of Japan, have the lowest occurrence of heart disease in the world—one-fifth that of the United States. Occurrence of breast, ovarian, and prostate cancer are significantly lower than that of the United States too. There are six times as many one-hundred-year-old people per capita there as in America. The world's longest disability- free life expectancies are also in Okinawa.

The people of Okinawa have a strong sense of community with high levels of social contact. Prayers are often about health. Health and longevity are celebrated, and the elderly are respected and considered wise. There are also extremely low levels of negative emotions and depression. In Okinawa, the diet of the islanders is:

Vegetables (Soy, leafy greens, etc.)	46 %
Whole grains	32 %
Fruit	6 %
Fish	11 %
Misc. (red meat, eggs, poultry)	5 %

That means that 95 percent of the diet of the healthiest humans in the world consists of various vegetables, whole grains, fish and fruit.

In his book *Blue Zones*, Dan Buettner tells the stories of three communities of elderly who reside in completely different parts of the world. The book was a follow-up to an article that appeared in the November 2005 issue of National Geographic entitled "New Wrinkles on Aging".

The communities of Sardinia, Italy have things in common with the communities of Okinawa; as well as the Seventh Day Adventist communities of Loma Linda, California. All three have a proportionately higher number of people one hundred years old or older compared to the rest of the world. *What do these three communities have in common?* All three have the following similarities: no smoking, family as first priority, active physical lifestyle, socially engaging communities, and healthy diets. Even though the three populations represent different regions and religions, all of them have diets that are dominated by fruits, vegetables, and whole grains.

Sardinians are shepherds. Okinawans are fisherman and farmers. Seventh Day Adventists of Loma Linda (the healthiest Americans) actively serve in various positions throughout the city. All three communities have very physical lifestyles.

A sad truth about each population is that some threads of traditions are being broken among the generations. The taste for fast food, the use of automobiles instead of walking or bicycling, using television and other electronic media are quickly becoming the preferred alternatives to the traditional, especially for the younger generations. With the increase of western diets, there is an increase in obesity and related illnesses. With this increase, there is the natural progression of *fad diet* solutions being sold.

Fad Diets vary considerably. It is reasonable to say that you could find a rationale to support any diet that you like; high carbohydrates, low carbohydrates and high protein, low fat, strictly calorie counting, diets that target blood type, vegetarian diets, and starvation diets. Some diets require supplements, powders, or specific food combinations; others are a matter of strict food control with no required supplementation.

With all these choices to try to confuse, regulate, or reduce our consumption; it is easy to forget that calorie intake is essential for sustaining life. We use calories from our diets throughout a normal day. Tampering too much, one way or the other, with caloric intake disrupts the body's natural need to stay in balance. Every day the body needs a certain number of calories, depending on one's size and activity level. When a large number of calories is taken away from a balanced diet, the body has an increased risk of losing muscle mass (or size). A smaller reduction of calories from a balanced diet with increased activity tends to make a more lasting body fat loss.

Starting as a war effort in May of 1941, the idea of Recommended Daily Allowances (RDA) for nutrients was introduced at the National Nutrition Conference to be a yardstick for identifying a standard of nutrition. People who did not take in those recommended allowances were identified as 'under-nourished'. Gradually, under-nourishment became a national focus. As a result, processed foods, such as white bread, became "fortified" or enriched with vitamins and minerals; and the food supplement industry exploded. Since then, RDAs have been revised and updated continuously. Look at the nutrition label on any bottle, can, or package of food you buy. The United States Food and Drug Administration (USDA) developed a comprehensive standard in nutritional values. "Daily Values" (DV) are currently based on a 2,000-calorie diet, although this is always being updated as new discoveries unfold in research. The total calories and the percentages recommended for fats, proteins, and carbohydrates are part of the nutrition label. Also included are sodium, fiber, vitamins, and minerals. This system is designed for the nutritional needs of average healthy adults, and is easily referred to on every food container. However, the system is not intended to tell individuals exactly what they need to eat each day.

Let's look a little more closely at each nutrient. I think the most important observation we can make when we look at an individual nutrient is not to discover what we 'have' to eat to satisfy the requirement, but how little the amount of healthy food we really need to satisfy the minimum requirement. Again, all values are subject to change depending on the latest research, but for now, these are the standards that have been around for a long time.

Proteins: The FDA recommends that 50 grams of protein be eaten on a daily basis in a 2,000-calorie diet. To better understand what 50 grams of protein is, one handful of peanuts (or 1/4 cup) is about seven grams, while two ounces of tuna fish is 14 grams. It doesn't take much to get to 50 grams in a day, if you eat healthy foods that are rich in protein. Heavy weight lifting activity and a body with a larger muscle mass increases one's need for protein. Lean (low-fat) proteins are found in almost all seafood, poultry, beans, and dark green vegetables. Nuts and seeds also have high concentrations of proteins, but with higher fat and calorie content. Again, it doesn't take much healthy food to reach 50 grams of protein in a day.

Carbohydrates: The FDA recommends that up to 300 grams of carbohydrates be consumed in a 2,000-calorie a day diet. A large whole-wheat bagel is 55 grams of carbohydrates, while eight ounces of regular orange juice has 26 grams. It is obvious that these numbers add up fast, especially with a diet of heavily processed fast foods and prepackaged food products.

Carbohydrates can raise blood sugar levels immediately by converting quickly to glucose and entering the bloodstream. When the blood sugar (glucose) level rises, so does the release of insulin from the pancreas. The more insulin released into one's system due to the intake of carbohydrates, the less stored body fat will be used for energy.

Diabetes is the condition of the pancreas not being able to produce enough insulin, or any at all. Excessive insulin in the blood can block the burning of fat for energy, making it more difficult to lose body fat with exercise. But it is important to understand that not all carbohydrates are created equal. Much of the carbohydrate found in vegetables, fruits, and whole grains is "dietary fiber". Dietary fiber is the part of the plant that cannot be digested. Even though dietary fiber is a carbohydrate; it does not cause a rise in blood sugar or a release of insulin. The FDA recommends at least 25 grams of fiber daily in a 2,000-calorie diet. Refined sugars and processed flours are the carbohydrates of the plants, fruits, and grains with the fiber removed. This process of refining leaves only the portion of carbohydrates that causes insulin to be released.

Glycemic Index: In the last decades of the 20th century and into this century, "The Glycemic Index" has become a very popular and useful dietary tool with the help of diet programs such as *Jenny Craig®, Nutri-System®,* and *Weight-Watchers®*; as well as, diets like *The Atkins Diet®, the Zone Diet®, the South Beach Diet®, SugarBusters®,* and many others. This index can help determine the effect that a certain food has on the blood and the food's effect on the release of insulin. Each particular food is compared to glucose, which has an assigned value of 100. All foods with carbohydrates will affect the insulin level. *The Glycemic Index* value of foods can be used to compare foods such as fruits and vegetables in their natural state to those that have been processed. The bottom line is that the more *whole* the food (the less it is processed), the lower the *Glycemic Index* number. Which means, the healthier it is for digestion and the slower release of insulin. This is primarily due to the dietary fiber content that remains in the food. Whole foods ensure the healthy fiber that was intended for a balanced diet. Fiber regulates the function of the digestive system, curbs hunger, and helps in the elimination of bacteria and cholesterol in the intestines. This is accomplished without added digested calories, increase of blood sugars, or a release of insulin. Whole foods, and especially their fiber, offer health benefits without added calories.

To put it another way, if one were to drink apple juice, almost 100 percent of the carbohydrates of that juice are carbohydrates that cause a rush of insulin to the bloodstream, thus blocking the body's ability to use stored fat for energy. If one ate the same serving as applesauce, 89 percent of the carbohydrates would affect insulin, 11 percent would not. With a whole apple, 82 percent of overall carbohydrates would affect insulin, 18 percent would not. This 18 percent is a different type of healthy fiber, which aids in digestion while not adding digested calories to the overall daily caloric intake. Eating a real apple greatly reduces the assigned Glycemic Index number, putting less strain on the pancreas to release large volumes of insulin into the blood at one time. The healthiest way to eat the apple is directly from the tree. Carbohydrates from strained orange juice affect insulin 100 percent. A whole orange is 79 percent carbohydrates affecting insulin and nearly 21 percent being healthy types of fiber. The same is true for wheat. Most white bread has about 5 percent fiber, while wheat bread has 10 percent fiber. This significantly decreases the release of insulin released from the pancreas, as well as, reduces the Glycemic Index number. The less processed the natural food; the better (or lower) the Glycemic Index number.

So, the Glycemic Index can be a valuable tool for determining which foods to eat in order to ensure healthy, slower, and lower release of insulin. But the simple rule of thumb is: the more real, whole, and less processed the food, with few exceptions, the healthier it is. This is the way it has been for thousands of years and still is today.

Fats: Some fat is necessary for keeping tissues in good repair, for manufacturing many hormones, and also for transporting some fat-soluble vitamins. The RDA for total fat is less than 65 grams (based on a 2,000-calorie diet). The most useful fats are found in fish and polyunsaturated oils from plants, such as olive, canola, and flaxseed oils.

Even though some fats are useful and they do not affect the blood sugars causing the release of insulin; they are not completely out of the woods. Fats are always high in calories and don't add a tremendous amount of nutrition beyond the small amount that you can get from one or two tablespoons of cod liver oil, five ounces of walnuts, or an avocado each day. Remember, to burn away body fat, you need to be aware of total calories. Fatty foods, even healthy ones, can add empty calories fast.

"Good" fats can be found in real foods, such as fish and nuts. "Bad" fats are the saturated fats found in butter, meats, and dairy products. Even worse are the fats that we have created ourselves. These are found in margarine and many other processed foods, such as potato chips and doughnuts. These are the trans-fatty acids.

Vitamins and Minerals: With few exceptions, all essential vitamins and minerals are found in whole grains, nuts, fruits, and vegetables, specifically leafy greens. The greater the variety of vegetables, fruits, nuts, and beans you consume, the healthier your overall diet. The greater the variety of whole foods you consume, the more essential vitamins and minerals your body will take in. Also, eating vitamins and minerals in their natural form, from healthy foods rather than from supplements, allows the digestive system to utilize them more efficiently. Such eating also reduces the risk of artificially ingesting an excess of any particular vitamin or mineral, which could lead to other problems such as blood poisoning or kidney stones.

Also, the National Cancer Institute supports five servings of vegetables and fruit daily for the reduction of several types of cancers. Marion Nestle, the chairperson of the Department of Nutrition, Food Studies, and Public Health at New York University said this in her book *Food Politics* regarding whole foods:

> "As an academic nutritionist, I grapple on a daily basis with what I see as a central contradiction between nutrition theory and practice. On the one hand, our advice about the health benefits of diets based largely on food plants—fruits, vegetables, and grains—has not changed in more than fifty years and is consistently supported by ongoing research. On the other hand, people seem increasingly confused about what they are supposed to eat to stay healthy. As a population, Americans are eating more animal-based foods—and more food in general—to the point where half of us are overweight, even our children are obese, and diseases related to diet are leading causes of death and disability."

Consider the story of Daniel in the Old Testament. When Daniel was appointed by the king of Babylon to his royal service, he was given the same diet of all the people of the palace. His rations were to be that of the wealthy, royal diet of rich food and wine. As with all prosperous kings' tables at the time, royal rations meant nothing but the finest fatted calves and pork, and much of it. Daniel suggested to the palace master to let him have only vegetables and water to eat while the rest of the royal servants ate the heavy animal-based foods from the royal table. The palace master, who feared the king, was afraid of the effects that only vegetables and water would have on Daniel. But Daniel talked him into a contest of ten days allowing him to eat only vegetables and water, while everyone else ate the rich foods and drank fine wine (probably the first documented weight-loss challenge). After ten days, Daniel was remarkably healthier than those who ate the fatty foods. So much so that the palace master ordered the vegetable diet for all the servants of the royal palace.

> *"I eat to live, to serve, and also, if it so happens, to enjoy, but I do not eat for the sake of enjoyment."*
> *-Mahatma Gandhi*

There is a phenomenon that is noted in research regarding affluence and nutrition. Marion Nestle calls this the "nutrition transition". As emerging nations become more and more prosperous, they tend to leave the dominant plant-based diets for more animal-based diets complete with heavy processing, refined sugars and flours, and lots of animal fat. This, of course, starts the cycle of rapid weight gain and chronic disease. The irony is that if the individuals were to continue with the plant-based rations, they would be much better off physically in spite of being a "prosperous" nation. The American diet contains huge quantities of refined sugars, processed flours, and heavy animal fats. It is obvious that such a diet was never intended for human consumption on a regular basis.

Volume: It is surprising how filling a diet rich in vegetables, fruit, and whole grains can be. You may also be shocked at the enormous volume of food you actually need to eat with a primarily plant-based diet as opposed to a highly processed, animal-based diet.

In her book <u>Volumetrics</u>, Elizabeth Bell, Ph.D. of Pennsylvania State University found that healthy women instinctively ate around the same volume or amount of food a day and it didn't matter whether it was high or low in calories. The weight of the food in a day remained the consistent amount; the quantity of food, and not the calories, satisfies one's desire to eat. In other words, if we ate equal amounts of healthy whole foods of lower calories with more nutrients in a day, we would more likely satisfy our desire long-term than if we were to eat less volume of unhealthy, processed, higher calorie foods.

Fruits and vegetables, like us humans, are made up of primarily water, which adds tremendous volume with no extra calories (we will discuss this in detail in the next chapter). Food volume might also be some insight as to why diets usually end up broken after a period of time. The desire for a certain amount of food instinctively overrides the desire to lose weight. To learn to eat and be filled with larger amounts of whole foods, might make certain a lifetime of proper nutrition and will naturally battle obesity in the long run.

Studies in the American Journal of Clinical Nutrition reveal that drinking sugar-rich drinks, such as regular soda, did not curb the appetite of a person throughout the day. Those drinking non-caloric drinks and those drinking sugar-rich drinks ate the same volume of food. It is clear that drinking sugar rich drinks will add to obesity by adding extra calories, but doing nothing to the overall desire for the volume of food in a day.

The conclusion is to not waste your calories in a day on things like sugar-rich drinks, high calorie *lattes,* or processed low nutrition foods. Save calories and volume of food for healthy, low-calorie, fiber-rich, whole food that will satisfy cravings by eating all you want. This will satisfy overall hunger and nutritional needs.

Nutrient Density: Dr. Fuhrman, M.D., author of *Eat to Live*, coined a wonderful formula. It determines the Nutrient Density of food choices. The formula says that health is equal to the nutrients you eat divided by the calories:

$$Health = Nutrients \div Calories$$

Simply put, the more nutrient-rich foods we eat that are low in calories, the better our health. Vegetables, which have extremely high nutrients for low calories, fit Dr. Fuhrman's formula very well. Fruit also has very high nutrients and fiber with enormous water content. Whole grains and beans are high in nutrients and fiber. Meats, refined sugars, and flours have lower overall nutrients and more calories. We can see that a diet rich in plant-based foods has greater nutrients and fewer calories than the animal-based and processed-food diets that are popular in America today.

We are overly trained about food do's and don'ts. But focusing on food choices, still keeps our attention on food. Striving for a balanced diet, Americans consume large amounts of vitamin supplements, prepackaged food bars, and nutritional shakes. Here, too, we have created so many things artificially to mimic what has been given to us naturally. A nutrition bar that has 320 calories could have a well-balanced set of nutrients and fiber. Ironically, you can eat about 110 asparagus spears to equal the same calories but with more protein, dietary fiber, vitamins A and C, calcium, iron, potassium, and with less fat and sodium. Eating 110 asparagus spears will certainly be more filling than a nutrition bar, just not quite as tasty. The same is true for green beans. Calories in one bar equal about ten cups of green beans; or with tomatoes, one bar equals about nine tomatoes. The calories from one nutrition bar equals four apples, three bananas, three pears, or eight cups of watermelon. All the mentioned fruits and vegetables have more fiber and less sodium and fat than that nutrition bar. Of course, this is a nutrition bar comparison to natural foods. Let's compare fast food with natural foods.

A Big Mac™, with 590 calories, is equal to about 190 asparagus spears. The burger has 34 grams of fat, while asparagus has zero. As you can see, it isn't that we do not have healthier choices; we just make different choices.

Living Water

Images of "living water" are used throughout all religions. In the gospel of John, Jesus describes himself as living water: "Those who drink of the water I will give him will never be thirsty" (John 4:14). The Samaritan woman to whom he speaks wished to know more about this water. She is shunned by the elite religious community as a Samaritan and also a sinner. It is not surprising that this hopeless women accepts Jesus' gift of living water, and begins to tell others about this life-changing drink.

In Thailand, there is a Buddhist festival called *Songkran* where folks gather at the riverbanks and release live fish into the river. The three day festival is marked with playful water splashing and celebration among villagers. The water symbolizes the washing away of all that is bad. Water cleanses the soul.

For Christians, baptism into new life is done with water. Rain is celebrated as life-giving. Throughout history, farmers have prayed for the one variable that can determine the difference between feast or famine—rain. Water is what sustains us and brings us life.

The human body is about 75 percent water. Blood is about 94 percent water. It is, without a doubt, an appropriate to talk of water as "life giving". Some researchers estimate that the changes in our diets from real fruits and vegetables to processed foods, and our higher consumption of diuretic drinks like soda, coffee, and alcohol have a clear negative dehydrating effect on our bodies. Real fruits and vegetables contain mostly water, like us humans. Alcohol and caffeine are diuretics that stimulate an increase in urine output. Processed foods are primarily dehydrated for better shipping and storage. We are a nation that is suffering from chronic dehydration. We lack "living water".

Water is not only important to every aspect of life, but it also aids digestion and adds bulk to food. Living things, like fruits and vegetables, all are sustained by and contain large quantities of water. The closer to the original version of the whole food, the more water it contains. Even though a raisin and a grape have equal calories, the water content makes the difference. The original form of the grape has much greater volume causing a feeling of satisfaction after eating the same amount of calories as the raisin. The grape has nearly eight times the volume or bulk than the raisin and with equal nutrients, plus grapes have a significantly lower Glycemic Index number than raisins.

When fresh whole fruits and vegetables come off the vine or tree and are eaten before any processing, they cause a more "full" feeling with equal calories than versions of the same fruit or vegetable that have either been dehydrated or stripped of their fiber.

In his book, *Water for Health for Healing for Life*, Dr. F. Batmanghelidj identifies forty-six reasons why the body needs ample water every day. The list includes water being the medium that transports all substances inside the body, its contribution to the prevention of obesity, and its role in decreasing joint and lower back pain.

Water is the source for all life. Lack of clean water is, and will continue to be, the most immediate threat to the lives of the very poor. By limiting the water we use for tasks that do not directly involve drinking or growing food (such as overwatering lawns); we not only save our own money, but we demonstrate compassion to our neighbors in our own neighborhood by better using our resources we share as a community.

Giving thanks for clean water is a wonderful practice. It reminds us to conserve and strive to make sure everyone has it. Such a life-giving gift must remain sacred so it can be shared.

One of the most powerful and important mission projects that can establish sustainability is the building of a village well that can bring water for drinking and for crops. A well can restore the gift of life.

When Henry David Thoreau spoke of diet, he mentioned that he eats only the simplest foods and refuses all alcoholic drinks because they might ruin his taste for water.

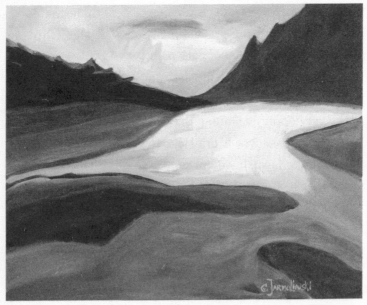

Acrylic painting entitled *Mountain Lake* by artist *Christina Jarmolinski*
www.jarmolinski.com

Price of Affluence

Are you ready to buy into the monumental shift from the current *need-to-lose-weight* way of thinking (or paradigm) to the *need-to-feed others* paradigm? We have already explored the fact that we are spending billions to help us curb our appetites while our neighbors have nothing. We realize the injustice of this, but what can we do about it? Looking a little deeper at this problem might help us move toward a life of our own health and wellness.

Do not underestimate your ability to initiate changes that make a real difference. Our efforts do not have to be so extreme. Supplying goods at the lowest cost possible to beat the competitor's prices for the consumer is what business does. When we, as consumers, make purchases based strictly on the cost or emotional desire, we may be inviting the evils of labor exploitation, deforestation, or unfair treatment of resources in order to get the lowest cost of a product. As consumers, we have to become transparent in our deeper desires through our purchases we make as we support those businesses that have been transparent and responsible with us, our neighbors, and our planet. Business, by design, will rise to meet the demands of the consumer. It is up to us, individually and collectively, to purchase goods that are offered with a social, environmental, and health consciousness. It is in our best interest and the best interest of our neighbors that we start to look past the attractive advertisements, and look more deeply into the truth of our own food consumption.

The United States Department of Agriculture (USDA) economists estimate that eating more fruit and vegetables and fewer foods of animal origin would upset the existing production of agricultural commodities and would require large "adjustments" in international food trade.

"Can America afford to switch its diet away from heavily processed, sugared, and animal-based diets to a more whole, natural, plant-based diet?" The question posed in this chapter is, *"Can America afford not to"*?

The average American child sees 10,000 food ads a year on television, and 95 percent of them are for sugared cereals, fast food, soft drinks, and candy. In 2010, Americans spent $137 billion on fast food. In 1970, that number was $6 billion. So, in 40 years there has been a 2283% increase in America's fast food spending. It is easy to see that our American diets have fundamentally changed and the secondary health and environmental problems have changed with it.

Garbage: Elizabeth Royte, the author of *Garbage Land* reminds us that for every ton of trash we throw away, there is considerably more "manufacturing and industrial" waste produced to make that product. Paper, plastic, tin, aluminum, and glass products are used directly through food processing and packaging. But there is also the behind the scenes manufacturing and industrial waste that is used to create each of those products.

Much can be done about the waste we produce with the foods we choose. A bag of fresh local fruit, vegetables, or legumes from the farmer's market could produce one reusable paper or plastic bag. The whole unprocessed food goes from harvest to the local consumer for sale. Processed foods run through a chain of conversions, travel, and middlemen until they eventually emerge as the product. Through the chain of conversions, there is an industrial waste that is produced along the way that outweighs the trash that is tossed out once the food product is unpacked. Processed foods produce both visible and hidden garbage.

Topsoil: Rich, healthy soil is disappearing through conventional farming techniques. I didn't fully understand this until I spent two years at the experimental farm at The Rodale Institute in Kutztown, Pennsylvania.

The Rodale Institute is a non-profit side of Rodale, Inc., which publishes popular wellness magazines like: *Prevention, Runner's, Bicycling, Organic Gardening*, and

Men's Health. The Rodale Institute's ongoing soil, farming, and produce research is showing how we are all affected by the farming industrial methods. The founder, J. I. Rodale, who originally coined the term *Organic*, was dedicated to the natural relationship we have to the soil. The Rodale Institute's motto is simple: *Healthy soil = Healthy food = Healthy people.*

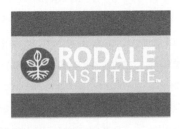

Since 1981, The Rodale Institute has been comparing organic and conventional grain-based farming systems. Through the use of heavy, conventional, manufactured fertilizers, herbicides, insecticides, and fungicides; our food, soil, and ecosystem have changed since the birth of the modern farming techniques after World War II. The research, which is now entering its fourth decade, reveals that by restoring nutrients to the soil naturally through organic methods of composting, crop rotations, cover crops, and more natural biodiversity; the farming environment is more apt to conserve soil, water, energy, and biological resources while adding nutrients to the crops. Modern farming does not rely on these natural techniques.

Composting adds a richer organic soil matter (carbon and nitrogen) which helps conserve water resources; and soil becomes more drought resistant. Employing natural biodiversity eliminates the need to use manufactured nitrogen fertilizers, herbicides, insecticides, and fungicides.

In essence, using farming techniques that have been around for six thousand years helps to restore the nutrients in the produce and in the environment. In a sense, it also provides stability for a farming future without manufactured fertilizers, herbicides, insecticides, fungicides, and tankers of fossil fuels that are required to manufacture those chemicals.

Visiting the Rodale farm is a powerful experience that cannot be communicated on paper. The farm concentrates on the soil as it was intended to be. When we take care of the soil, it will take care of us. The ongoing studies reveal something that someone of faith already knows: God provides naturally. We are called to be good stewards of the soil that we have been given.

In an era of fast food, it is extremely important that we take time to rediscover the spiritual value of food. Cultivate eating as an opportunity to express humble

gratitude for the abundance we experience in our lives. In addition, when we eat with those we are close to, eating has even special meaning far beyond calories and nutrients . . . savor that moment. "Dear Lord, thank you for this daily bread and all the efforts of those who have brought it to this table. Let me and mine be of Thy service. Amen."
—Paul Reed Hepperly, Ph.D.
   Research Manager, The Rodale Institute

When you walk around the 333-acre Rodale Institute farmland, you get a feeling of optimism. It is a realization that if people were given a chance, we would collectively right the wrongs of the way we treat our land because of our current appetites.

This same feeling of optimism is also present for similar reasons when you visit the ECHO demonstration farm in North Fort Myers, Florida.

ECHO *(Educational Concerns for Hunger Organization)* is a 55-acre laboratory that has a plethora of displays demonstrating living situations in the tropical Third World. ECHO's objective is to help those working internationally with the poor to be more effective, especially in the area of agriculture.

Some of the solutions to the problems that Third World countries face that are addressed at ECHO are: rooftop farming in heavily populated urban areas where ground is scarce; terracing where the natural terrain is not farmable; farming in rainforests, monsoon regions, and arid regions; and solutions to bad soil using natural resources. The mission of ECHO is solving problems. They offer possibilities that seem impossible, such as ways of trapping rainwater and planting using abandoned garbage. They educate missionaries to the 180 countries that are in desperate need of stable agriculture.

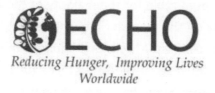

Reducing Hunger, Improving Lives
Worldwide

When you visit ECHO, you get that same feeling of hope that the Rodale Institute gives you. There is something so pure and spiritual about caring for the soil—that feeling of graciousness, knowing that we all live because of our nurturing relationship with the earth. When we do not experience this relationship, we run the risk of treating the planet like we are its demanding masters. We take and take and eventually run it out of business.

> God said, "See, I have given you every plant yielding seed that is upon the face of all the earth, and every tree with seed in its fruit; you shall have them for food."
> —Genesis 1:29

Cheap Meat: Since the great majority of the corn that is farmed in the United States goes to feed livestock (approximately 80 percent); it would make sense that livestock is responsible for the majority of the water that is used directly on the crops for growing. In fact, the majority of the water used from wells and aquifers in America does go to crops for feed. If the same crops (or other types of vegetables) were given directly to humans for consumption instead of livestock, the efficiency of food volume would be greatly increased. Vegetables, fruits, legumes, and whole grains eaten directly by humans create a great deal more volume of food compared to feeding it to cattle and then eating the meat. Likewise, the water used to produce the same volume of healthier food would go down significantly when compared to meat.

From one acre of land, roughly **250 pounds of beef** can be produced from the corn to the cattle. In that same acre of fertile soil, through the lifetime of the cattle before slaughter, you could produce any one of these vegetable amounts:

30,000 pounds of carrots, or
40,000 pounds of potatoes, or
40,000 pounds of onions, or
50,000 pounds of tomatoes, or
60,000 pounds of celery

Vegetables can be grown in a fraction of the space that is needed for the corn in order to feed the cattle for beef. It is estimated that the livestock in the United States eat enough corn and soybeans to feed the entire population of the country five times over.

High density feedlots create more meat in less space. But, the high volume of manure in a concentrated area causes both a soil imbalance and an increased need for antibiotics for the animals. Currently, we ingest more traces of animal antibiotics, pesticides, and fertilizers than sixty years ago. The demand has risen consistently for inexpensive meats over the past half century. It is the demand for unhealthy, cheap meats that has pushed commercial farmers to supply the current demand while staying at competitive prices.

Foreign Oil: In addition to degrading our soil, current conventional farming techniques have also consumed our fossil fuels at a higher rate than sixty years ago. With mass commercial farming and the large consumption of prepackaged processed foods, food products are grown miles from where they are sold. The journey begins in the fields, then to the processing plants, to packaging, and finally to the stores or fast food restaurants for the consumer. Fossil fuels are used at an enormous rates for the shipping of food and food products to different destinations. Fossil fuels are also used in greater concentrations to produce the conventional farming fertilizers, insecticides, and weed killers that organic farming does not.

Rain Forests: We have looked at how the current food market affects our country's natural resources. Now let's take a step back and look at a more global picture. An area of constant focus has been the rainforests.

The rainforests provide natural habitats to thousands of plant and animal species; as well as, help toward stabilizing global climate. But our world's rainforests are being destroyed at an astounding rate. Beyond all of the natural resources we lose as the rainforests shrink, that loss is also affecting the global climate.

The accumulation of heat-trapping gases (carbon dioxide and carbon monoxide) that are emitted from the burning of fossil fuels such as coal, oil, and gasoline; as well as, the reduction of overall trees and plant life in the world; causes the slow and steady heating of the earth's climate. Carbon dioxide becomes more prevalent the more fossil fuels are burned, the more artificial fertilizers are used on crops and the fewer trees there are. To simplify, humans breathe in air to utilize the oxygen, then exhale carbon dioxide. Trees and plants, for the most part, do the opposite. Trees utilize heat-trapping carbon dioxide and emit oxygen.

We were created to live in harmony with trees and plants; but the evidence suggests that the increased burning of fossil fuels and the destruction of the world's rainforests throws off the symbiosis of our ecosystem. The result is a slightly higher carbon-gas rich atmosphere that traps heat and causes the weather to warm-up globally. So, between having fewer trees, more burned fossil fuels, and heavy use of manufactured chemical fertilizers and pesticides; the natural state of the atmosphere is affected by the heavy demand of cheap meat.

The lumber from the rainforest is sold and the majority of the stripped land is used in other ways. Most of the land is used to grow corn and soy beans for livestock. As the demand for beef increases, so does the need for rich land for feed for the livestock. Seldom is there a large replanting effort to replenish the lost trees.

The native people live off the resources of the rainforest. Without the rainforests; people, animals, and plants lose. In addition to reducing the effects of global warming, the rainforests need to be protected for the natural resources they provide the indigenous people who rely on their vegetation and canopy.

Healthy shifts toward sustaining and replenishing the resources which are harvested directly from what already exists in the rainforests (medicinal plants, natural fruit, nuts, rubber products, shade grown coffee, and cocoa beans) would help the ecosystem of our neighbor's land survive. Income for those poorer countries could be based on the sustainable natural resources that already exists. There would be no need to strip the land.

Some companies, like *Ben & Jerry's Homemade, Inc.*, have raised public awareness of the shrinking rainforests and have become proactive in the battle to save them by using the natural resources that the rainforests provide (vanilla extract, cashews, and Brazilian nuts). Shade grown coffee, tea, and cocoa are bought and traded through the Equal Exchange food co-op; as well as, eco-friendly companies.

These organizations and others like it supply farmers with a fair market, offer a consistent price for their products, and maintain the natural resources by leaving ecosystems intact such as supporting the growth of "shaded" organic coffee. This shaded coffee grows in its natural environment without the use of chemical fertilizers and pesticides. The International Fair Trade Association is a good resource that networks socially, environmentally, and medically sound organizations together with consumers who don't base their purchases on cost alone, but on the overall global value as well. If goods are purchased carefully, all boats (not just yachts) will rise with the tide.

Feed My Sheep

In 1963, President John F. Kennedy stated to congress, "We have the ability, we have the means, and we have the capacity to eliminate hunger from the face of the earth in our lifetime. We need only the will".

More recently, in 2006, Jeffrey D. Sachs the author of *The End of Poverty* made clear that extreme poverty could be eliminated forever with the involvement of the global community.

This might be a good place to mention a commonly held misconception related to global poverty. People ask, *"Doesn't starvation keep the populations down in those countries that are overpopulated anyway? If we feed everyone, won't the global population just grow to an unmanageable number?"*

To answer frankly, absolutely not! Poverty is what causes overpopulation in the Third World. A population's growth cycle decreases and stabilizes in developing countries as families receive real opportunities.

The populations of thriving, developed countries typically have a steady number of births and deaths. In recent years, populations have actually shown a sharp decline in the wealthy nations. Underdeveloped countries—countries with limited government infrastructures—like schools, electricity, maintained roads, and healthcare— have considerably more children born per mother. We can trace these trends in birth rate directly to several factors, and all of them have to do with poverty.

- First of all, impoverished children die in larger numbers than children with financial means. Women give birth to many more children to compensate for the increased infant mortality.
- Secondly, as a society moves from an agricultural base to urban settings, the need for many children diminishes. Upgraded farming equipment and stable working conditions mean families need the labor of fewer children.
- Third, improved healthcare leads to more surviving infants, greatly reducing the need and desire for more pregnancies. Healthcare also introduces careful family planning methods.
- Finally, education! The more access women have to education—learning about trades, reproductive choices, and good health—the fewer children are born. Parents who can choose the size of their families will have the time and energy to invest in their children along with a commitment to their education. Families simply get smaller.

"All of these factors (jobs, careful family planning, healthcare and education) explain why most of the world has achieved a marked reduction of total fertility rates and a sharp slowdown in population growth."

-Jeffrey Sachs, The End of Poverty

With a disciplined consciousness about our eating and with a compassion for our hungry neighbors; we will solve the epidemic of obesity and the shameful imbalance of world hunger, control the population explosions of the Third World, and move away from further destruction of our environment. This is truly "food for thought".

Eating differently for the benefit of our own health, our neighbor's health, and the environment sounds ambitious— and it is. Never the less, the choices we privileged consumers make have awesome consequences. In reality, it can be done with little effort on our part.

Ninety Percent Produce

A simple idea we can adopt towards a more balanced healthy diet for ourselves as well as our neighbors and the planet is to start working towards eating a more locally grown "ninety percent produce diet". Our diet can mimic that of Okinawa's villagers, the healthiest people on the planet.

Compared to a current heavy animal-based processed diet, a majority plant-based diet, which is 90% of the overall calories in a day, should consist of a variety of vegetables, fruits, whole grains, beans, nuts, and seeds. Following this guideline would reduce the risk of the following: *obesity, heart disease, hypertension, stroke, diabetes, certain cancers, and run-a-way healthcare costs.*

Because most food currently travels an average of thirteen hundred miles from the farm, through the processing factories, and to the consumer; our carbon footprint would be reduced exponentially if our ninety percent produce diet were predominantly local, seasonal, and organic produce. If we work towards this the following would happen: *dependency on fossil fuels would reduce, pollution would decline, local small farms would be supported, and community supported agriculture (CSA) would increase.*

Also, eating this way, would greatly effect the garbage produced (The 4.5 pounds of garbage per human that's produced each day could potentially be reduced up to 90%). The organic skins, peels, and shells from the produce eaten can be directly returned to enrich the soil through composting in a personal, church, or community garden.

The majority of the overall drinkable water used today goes directly to the fields to grow feed for livestock. Changing the nation to a predominately plant based diet from an animal-based diet would be one of the single most effective ways to conserve drinkable water (our most precious and disappearing resource). High-density feedlots would decline, while rainforest destruction would diminish due to less demand for cattle grazing, commercial feed corn, and soy bean production.

The current American diet, with over half of the daily calories coming from animal products (beef, poultry, cheese, eggs, and dairy), could be improved considerably with personal health, weight loss, and environmental benefit by replacing the animal-based foods with plant-based, non-processed, and locally grown foods such as: leafy green vegetables, fruits, nuts, seeds, beans, and whole grains. Michael Pollan dedicated the entire 250 plus pages of his 2009 book *In Defense of Food* to that thought. Pollan's conclusion to improve our personal health is boiled down to this: "Eat Food. Not too Much. Mostly Plants".

Dean Ornish, the famous Cardiologist and author, agrees with his colleagues that a simple diet that steers clear of animal fats and processed sugars, along with steady exercise, would reduce the chronic conditions of our nation's population by 95%. This would practically erase premature death by heart disease, type II diabetes, hypertension, risk of stroke, and certain cancers.

There is some great news developing throughout America. Nationally, there has been a sharp increase in numbers of organic family farms reappearing around the country. Community supported Agriculture and local Farmer's Markets have exploded in popularity since the first print of this book in 2006. The USDA reports that the number of Farmer's Market's rose from 1,755 in 1998 to 5,274 in 2009, and it continues to grow quickly. The Community Supported Agriculture (CSA) is even growing faster. Even though this counter-culture of simple whole foods existed along side the conventional food systems in America for many years (probably since the 1970s), it has recently picked up momentum as more and more Americans become disenchanted with the shortcomings of the health of the modern conventional food systems.

As stated before, the United States Department of Agriculture (USDA) economists estimate that eating more fruit and vegetables and fewer foods of animal origin would upset the existing production of agricultural commodities, and would require large "adjustments" in international food trade.

"Can America afford to switch its diet away from heavily processed, sugared, and animal-based diets to a more whole, natural, plant-based diet?" The question is posed again, "Can America afford not to"?

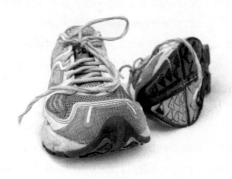

Exercise

Unlike anything we create by hand, like a car or a refrigerator which starts to breakdown when used, the body improves in every way with moderate to heavy use. Exercise is a magic pill, a fountain of youth, an anti-depressant. The body is improved in every way possible, naturally with exercise. The Creator intended for us to move and move a lot for optimum health by design.

"We have found the fountain of youth: it's exercise. Think about how you will be living the last twenty years of your life. Exercise today will have a tremendous effect on those years. The magic of the fountain of youth is that it keeps you younger even as you get older".
—Covert Bailey, The New Fit or Fat

You are unique. You never were before. You never will be again. You are wonderfully created with certain quirks, habits, interests, hobbies, and most importantly, gifts to offer the world—truly unique gifts that only you can give.

Of this I'm sure: we cannot fully explain the miracle that is us. We are beyond words. The language we use to describe the body speaks of "systems" and "cells", but we are limited in our full understanding. We speak of diseases in old age, but we miss the miracle and wonder of many years of perfectly good health. We are carefully planned, thought through in every loving detail. The human body is wonderfully made; it is God's greatest creation. In our search for miracles, one needs only peer under one's own skin to see the greatest of miracles; the miracle of life!

We are shooting in the dark when we explain life without the intelligent design of a careful and creative Creator. A

Creator who is both intentional and loving. We are not the result of chance.

> *"Only petty minds and trivial souls yearn for supernatural events, incapable of perceiving that everything—everything!—within and around them is pure miracle."*
> -Edward Abbey

To view the inner workings of that rarely-seen world that is inside the human body, the medical student can only stand and marvel as he learns. That is, if he does not miss the forest as he studies the trees. It has become my deepest passion to teach others to care for the greatest tool for which they have been gifted—their own body. The body in which they are entrusted to be a good steward of during their lifetime. With care, it will be animated for a hopeful one-hundred years and then returned to the elements in which it came.

We are no genetic mistake. We are made for significance, carefully created and intricately detailed. As spiritual beings, we can make the best of the temporary earthly journey we are all on together.

We are capable. Our minds can imagine, reason, and create. *Below* that, we have the capacity for the most remedial of tasks. But yet those trivial tasks require the depth of detail that only an intelligence beyond our comprehension could have intended.

The simple movement of a leg muscle requires an absolute orchestra of chemicals and electrical charges, carefully timed and choreographed. Simultaneous "inhibition" of the opposing muscles needs to be timed appropriately-opposing muscles lengthening only at a perfect rate so these muscles will not tear under tension...think about that...and this is only the abridged version of the muscular system functioning during a single leg muscle contraction. While this goes on, every other system in the body cooperates to make it happen. It is easy to overlook a miracle when it is you.

Now it is time for a second shift in thinking or paradigm shift. To review, in the food chapter, we discussed the shift from current "need-to-lose weight" model toward a "need-to-feed others" model. With this thinking, this nation would lose weight more easily. More importantly, we would feed the poor. This *second* shift in thinking is to see *exercise* as the gift it is. Exercise is a gift that will manifest in us a healthy long life. We should no longer see exercise as the chore we had made it to be. We can *care for ourselves to better care for others,* through the discipline of exercise.

Aging: At the <u>Gulf Coast Village Retirement Community</u> in Southwest Florida, you can find Charlie Crossen walking the 33 acre campus every morning before the heavy heat of the day. His long walks clear his head, strengthen his muscles, and continue to keep his heart and lungs healthy. Charlie had his 101st birthday recently and shows no signs of slowing down. Exercise is something he has done his entire life and has no desire to stop now. He often jokes to the visiting passerby that the reason he goes out for his daily walks is so he can 'chase the girls' who might also be out walking.

During WWII, Charlie was responsible for the fueling of the Navy war ships along the east coast of the United States. He had a significant responsibility better than seventy years ago. He still sees his life of having considerable significance.

Not far from Charlie at the *Sports Medicine and Wellness Center*, Rudy prepares to complete his second of three sets on the leg press. Rudy has just turned ninety-eight years old. He has deliberately exercised every day so that he can remember. At eighty years old, he had to quit running because it started to be hard on his arthritic right knee. Eighteen years later, he continues to do strength training and walking. Rudy feels that you need to work out with consistency or else 'you can't move at all'. He would say "You get rusty if you don't exercise every day". Rudy always ate healthy from the farm. He never picked up unhealthy habits like excessive drinking, smoking, or the taste for fast food.

Rudy and Charlie are thankful for every day. Rarely do they speak of their own struggles or pain even though they exist. Being "contented" is a conscious choice. It is refusing to be self-absorbed in one's own limitations or self-pity. Their disciplined physical life of exercise and healthy habits had only deepened their spiritual health.

"We have found the fountain of youth: it's exercise". The body is a miracle; it can heal and strengthen with a disciplined exercise program that addresses aging problems and fitness. Adhering closely to exercise and proper nutrition will increase the chances for an individual to remain disability-free until the end of life.

The majority of the body's decline is due not to the passing of years, but to the combined efforts of inactivity, poor nutrition, and illness, much of which can be controlled. Regardless of age or present physical condition, the aging process can be slowed and—often times—even reversed.

Rigorous exercises and physical work do not break down muscle, bone, heart, and lungs; but builds them up.

Movement improves the body's efficiency. In the book *Successful Aging*, a ten-year study uncovered a solid truth of aging: declining physical function is preventable and reversible.

We see the significance of exercise. It has the ability to change us completely. We become more efficient in everyway. Because of this, the deeper things in life that matter most can only be enhanced through fitness.

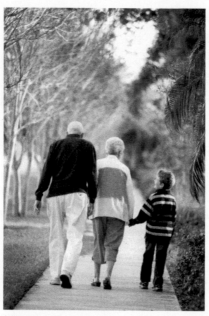

(photo: www.MelindaHawkins.com)

Healthcare: Today, healthcare costs are approaching 20 percent of the Gross National Product (GNP). The percentage of spending continues to increase at a faster rate as more Americans become dependent on medications and procedures that medical experts feel that 95% of these chronic diseases could be prevented through a lifestyle of proper diet and exercise.

As we learned in the food chapter, we are spending roughly 13 percent of all our GNP in America or about one trillion dollars on food and the food industry. The estimate is that about 3,800 calories are produced daily per person in America with this expense. This is almost twice the number of calories we need! If we add our healthcare costs and our food costs together (about 17.6 percent and 13 percent respectively), we can see that for every dollar spent in America, more than thirty cents goes to food and health care.

Knowing what we know regarding the chronic conditions mentioned: arthritis, osteoporosis, heart disease, hypertension, depression, and diabetes, what role might exercise play in reducing the run-a-way costs of prescription medications and treatment for chronic conditions?

Without question, exercise has a role in slowing the development of almost all early disability or life threatening ailments. The single most important step we can take as a nation to secure our healthcare system is to start eating healthier and exercising faithfully today and everyday after.

Arthritis: Osteoarthritis (generally called arthritis) is the name for the typical wearing away of the cartilage on the bone surfaces to the point of damage. Eventually, there is "bone on bone" and pain receptors are triggered. People with arthritis do not experience smooth movement of the joints. This causes creaking or "crepitus" in those joints. This is the point in typical arthritis when it is tough to move the joint without discomfort. If the knee or hip joint is affected, walking becomes very difficult. When arthritis gets to the stage in which even pain or anti-inflammatory medications no longer help, then a surgeon might opt for a total joint replacement to restore function to the patient.

This is a typical scenario for most senior citizens. Arthritis happens. A joint cannot stay young forever. However, it is interesting to see that individuals who have been consistent with exercises for years, have remained ambulatory with minimal pain even late into their nineties.

In the early stages of arthritis pain (let's say, age sixty), you may start to get a little "catch" or pain in the knee. You notice it most often after a long car ride or first thing in the morning. Instinctively, you start to favor that knee. You stop walking as long as you used to or not push it quite as hard as before in fear that there is something wrong with it. You think that someday you should get it 'checked-out'; but you don't, and you just live with it. Years go by and one of two things happened: either it cleared up on its own, or the pain had made it difficult to walk. Sometimes joint pain does go away—primarily because of the way joint surfaces get nutrition. But cartilage, which is the lining surface of the joint as well as padding between the bones, has a poor blood supply. Because of this, it doesn't get fed its nutrients as do other tissues of the body, like muscles, that have a good blood supply. Cartilage gets its nutrients from fluid (synovial fluid inside the joint) exchange. It is actual joint movement that allows the joint to rejuvenate itself. Compressive forces of the joint rebuilds and repairs itself while restoring the joints flexibility. The process can be compared to working taffy. When taffy is cold and dormant, it is hard and brittle; but when you start to pull it or "exercise" it, it becomes moldable or pliable. The pain you first feel might cause you to not move the joint much for fear that something is wrong; but movement is usually precisely what the joint needs for a consistent length of time.

If pain does not go away naturally with exercise, the joint cartilage itself could have been significantly damaged and in need of arthroscopic surgery by an orthopedic surgeon.

Exercising the joint to replenish with nutrients should almost always be the first conservative treatment choice. A good orthopedic surgeon will diagnose the difference between significant cartilage damage that requires surgery, and joint pain that could be treated with exercise.

When arthritis becomes significant and there is much difficulty walking, using a stationary bike will continue to ensure nutrient exchange to the joint, slowing the arthritic process without the painful weight-bearing of walking or running. Movement will help arthritis, especially in the early stages.

Osteoporosis: Without fail, exercise will help slow the progression of osteoporosis. The effects of weight-bearing exercises like walking or running cause an increase in the density of bone. The effectiveness is directly proportional to the intensity of the exercises. Weight lifting exercises will also help increase bone density. It has been shown to be as effective—if not more effective—than the use of prescription drugs for osteoporosis. However, clinical trials highlight the value of using exercise in conjunction with the prescription medications for the battle against advancing osteoporosis. The most effective prevention of osteoporosis is early rigorous exercise that includes weight-bearing and some sort of weight lifting (free weights, exercise bands, or weight machines). For women, exercise battles osteoporosis best if they are pre-menopausal; but post-menopausal women find benefit from exercise and osteoporosis prevention as well.

Heart Disease: The heart and lungs are strengthened with exercise. Typically, aerobic type exercise (walking, running, bicycling, swimming, etc.) works best to improve the condition of the cardiovascular and respiratory systems (heart, lungs, blood vessels, and blood). Aerobic activity stimulates the oxygen exchange of all the organs and encourages healing in any part of the body. What is considered aerobic activity? An easy rule of thumb when you are exercising is: if you can talk in a short sentence without gasping, that is considered aerobic. If you can talk in long-sentence conversation without breathing heavily, the exercise level might not be challenging enough. Pick up the pace in order to get a maximum benefit of your aerobic efforts. If you gasp for breath at every word, you might be going too hard; slowing down in order to exercise for a longer time or distance would be more beneficial.

Destructive habits, like smoking, not only compromise breathing and make exercise difficult; but they can also negatively affect healing and increase pain following an injury. The more you improve your cardiovascular system through disciplined exercises and non-destructive habits; the better the rest of your body systems work, because of the key role your heart and lungs have on bringing oxygenated blood to all parts of the body.

Hypertension: Hypertension or high blood pressure often can be managed with exercise. As you exercise over time, the heart becomes more efficient at pumping a larger volume of blood per beat. Since hypertension is excessive pressure against the walls of the blood vessels throughout the body, the more efficiently the heart pumps or forces blood out with each contraction, the less constant tension there will be on the blood vessel walls to move the same amount of blood. Stress is also a risk factor for hypertension. The sympathetic nervous system is stimulated with stress. We have a heightened sensitivity in times of anxiety. This is helpful when we are in danger, but not when it is self-inflicted or the result of lifestyle choices. When we are stressed, blood flow is constricted to our digestive system to allow more blood for our muscular system—in case we need to fight or flee from danger. Among other things, stress causes an increase in blood pressure and heart rate. If stress is a way of life, one may be at risk for digestive problems, disturbed sleeping patterns, even stroke and heart attack. Long-term effects of disciplined exercise may decrease in the stress of daily life by improving the cardiac output; as well as, releasing natural chemicals that reduce anxiety.

Excessive body fat also puts more stress on the heart to pump. The less body fat one has, the less stress one has on the heart and blood vessels as they pump the same volume of blood through the body. So, exercise not only reduces body fat; but it will directly decreases the tension on the heart and blood vessel walls; therefore, moving blood more efficiently through the body. This, in turn, reduces hypertension.

Stroke: A stroke happens when part of the brain does not have rich oxygenated blood circulating to it. A stroke can be caused by a thrombosis in which plaque (fatty deposit) is built up inside the blood vessel and finally occludes or chokes off the blood to a particular part of the brain. It can also be caused by an embolism in which the blood vessel is blocked off from plaque that has formed elsewhere, broken free, and settled in the small blood vessels of the brain causing a blocking of the blood. Either way, that part of the brain will die. A third way a stroke happens is by a hemorrhage, in which a blood vessel in the brain bursts under pressure or at a weakened spot in the vessel wall causing blood to spill out of the vessel and kill the part of the brain that no longer gets blood delivered to it. In each case, the better the circulation, the more pliable the blood vessels; and the lower the blood pressure, the lower the risk of a stroke. Understand, that consistent exercise contributes positively to all of these things. Exercise improves circulation, makes blood vessels more pliable by reducing the buildup of plaque, and lowers blood pressure. Therefore, consistent exercise, especially aerobic exercise, reduces the risk of stroke.

Diabetes: Diabetes is a condition that affects millions. There are two types of diabetes: Type I and Type II. Type I, formally called juvenile diabetes, is the direct result of the pancreas not producing insulin. Type I usually starts in childhood and may be present at birth; but most often, is a result of an autoimmune reaction in which the pancreas is affected by a virus. In Type II diabetes, the pancreas produces too little insulin, or the body has built a resistance to insulin; and it is not as effective in using glucose (sugar) for energy from the cells. Type II diabetes represents 90 percent of all diabetes and is the one that has grown to epidemic proportions in the United States. This epidemic has been linked directly to extremely poor diets and sedentary lifestyles.

The bottom line is the following regarding diabetes: damage is done to the body when sugar levels in the blood are too high or last too long. This can lead to cardiac conditions, blindness, kidney failure, stroke, or infection resulting in amputation. Exercise is a natural way to bring blood sugars down.

When you are at rest, your body (muscles and heart) demands only a little sugar (glucose) to be used for energy. With exercise, the demand for sugar greatly increases in the muscles and blood-sugar levels come down if they were running high. A sedentary individual who never exercises, sometimes experiences blood-sugar levels that stay higher. When you add to this high-sugar condition an unhealthy diet of excessive carbohydrates like refined sugar and processed flour, the individual's blood-sugar will start to rise simply because the body becomes resistant to the excessive amounts of sugar in the blood. In other words, the insulin is no longer effective enough to keep up with all those excess carbohydrates and no other way to burn all that sugar in the blood. Exercise works incredibly well to counter this problem. As you increase the demand on the body, the blood-sugar levels come down. Healthy, exercised muscles have the capacity to rapidly select the fuel source they need, sugar or fat, during times of fasting or feeding. Untrained muscles or unexercised muscles are more insulin resistant— unable to use sugar efficiently for energy even with insulin present. Think of unexercised muscles as having less ability to use the energy source they have. That is why the more you exercise the better you are at utilizing calories—and the less likely you are to develop Type II diabetes or obesity.

A word of caution regarding exercise for Type I diabetics or Type II diabetics who have a pancreas that is unable to produce enough insulin: vigorous exercise is so efficient at burning off excessive sugar that it is easy to go below your normal, healthy blood-sugar level and produce a low blood-sugar condition while you exercise. For this reason, it is most important to know your sugar levels if you've been diagnosed with diabetes. You need to stabilize your sugars by using the right amount of exercise along with the right dosage of insulin and the right amount of food, specifically carbohydrates.

This information should be a wake-up call for those who have very poor diets, who are obese, and don't exercise. It is this group that is most at risk for developing Type II diabetes. If they consistently exercise and eat healthy, they will greatly reduce their risk by giving their pancreas a break from the diet it was never intended by nature to handle.

In addition to chronic conditions requiring medications, exercise addresses other aspects of aging in ways no other medication or activity can.

Posture & Flexibility: Along with strength, flexibility is also compromised with a sedentary lifestyle. Just by adding activity to an inactive lifestyle, general flexibility will improve; but specific muscle groups should be addressed as well. As we age, our posture typically changes, mostly due to the effects of gravity, sarcopenia, and osteoporosis. We develop rounded shoulders and a forward head posture due to loss of flexibility of the chest and neck muscles, while weakening the muscles that keep the spine and shoulder blades in an erect position. This causes the shoulders and neck to slump forward, changing the posture. Exercises, specifically strengthening exercises, can address these areas to make sure the postural muscles and the chest and neck muscles maintain their strength and flexibility.

Also, muscles of the hips and legs tend to lose flexibility with prolonged sitting or inactivity. It is important to maintain flexibility and strength of these areas to ensure correct posture and function. When you don't exercise, the muscles in the hips (hip flexors) become shortened because of excessive sitting. With exercise you get to use the muscles' full available range of motion. The same is true for the muscles in the back of the legs, the hamstrings. Sitting causes this group of muscles to shorten. Standing and exercising, allows these muscles to work through their full range of motion. Aerobic activity improves circulation and this also assists in giving the muscles back their normal flexibility.

Depression: Exercise also affects depression in a positive way. Addictive substances such as: alcohol, cocaine, and tobacco stimulate the areas of the brain that cause a craving for more, so does exercise. This is done through a neurotransmitter "Dopamine".

Exercise, once a routine, becomes a healthy stimulant that can satisfy addictive cravings. Destructive addictive habits are then replaced by exercise, the healthy alternative. Exercise functions like an anti-depressant. So, the more you exercise, the more you desire to exercise and the less depressed you feel. Along with improved strength, endurance, flexibility, balance, and reduced risk of osteoporosis and sarcopenia; the benefit of reduced levels of depression is also a benefit with consistent exercise.

Metabolism: A closer look at the effects of exercise and diet can help us better understand their involvement in battling obesity and related chronic conditions. It is time to forget the breakthrough diet and self-help books, the new improved exercise programs and gadgets, the easy diet pill, and new food discoveries. What's true today has always been true: If today, you eat less calories than you burned-up, then you will lose weight, today. The same is true for tomorrow. Success of any diet will boil down to that relationship. The caloric intake cannot consistently exceed the calorie output. Simple physiology dictates that you will gain weight if input is greater than output consistently, whether the calories are proteins, fats, or carbohydrates. Your body will either store useful calories away for tomorrow, or burn them for energy today.

More muscle-More calories: Weight loss through exercise is affected by overall muscle size. Quite simply, the more muscle you have, the easier it is to burn fat. Muscle burns calories and fat does not. Plain and simple, fat cannot burn calories. Fat *is* stored calories. Aerobic conditioning and weight lifting both will burn calories. The calories burned in an exercise routine are directly proportional to the amount of muscle or lean body mass that you have. The calorie is actually a measurement of heat. The bigger your engine, the more potential you have to produce heat. Better put . . . the bigger the fireplace (muscle), the more wood (calories) you can burn at one time.

After weight lifting, your body uses extra calories to "grow" the muscle that you just exercised. Muscle growth (hypertrophy) utilizes extra calories following a workout. After a weight training session, "micro-tears" in the muscles happen. This is a normal occurrence. During the next couple of days, proteins help to repair and rebuild the muscles longer than before. A bigger "engine" results. This takes calories.

As stated before, calories must come from a well-balanced diet. This is most important to remember when you are trying to build a bigger engine. Weight lifting and starvation will never work together. If you really want to lose body fat, you need to create a bigger engine and burn more calories all day long; even while you sleep.

Weight lifting—whether using dumbbells, exercise bands, or machines—is a vital component of an exercise program to maintain current muscle mass. If done correctly and with the right intensity, weight lifting can truly reverse the natural aging process by maintaining or even growing the muscles that shrink (sarcopenia) with aging.

Slow and Steady: If you lose weight too rapidly, you can lose muscle as well. When high physical demands are put on a body that is in a "starvation" mode, the body retrieves extra calories for energy from proteins in the muscles and other places as well as stored fat. This is why when you starve and exercise, you cannot expect optimum results. The effects of this can be seen with individuals who deny themselves food but also have an insatiable need to exercise excessively, as with "Anorexia Nervosa". Since a young person's body needs energy for growing, it searches out any calories it can find to feed the obsession and can damage various systems of the body in the process.

If you average approximately 500 calories burned (used) daily with exercise, you will burn 3,500 calories extra each week with exercise. This means losing approximately one pound of fat per week, if calorie intake remains constant. One or two pounds a week of body fat lost is to be the safest and most permanent pace to lose weight.

Some people have a tendency to gain body fat more quickly than others; but it still holds true that it takes excess calories to create additional body fat. A tendency to gain body fat or a difficulty reducing body fat is often referred to as having a "slow metabolism". A slow metabolism is often a result of low activity of the body's systems, primarily the muscular system. A high metabolism is typically due to high activity. So metabolism reflects the number of calories that have been expended or burned in a day. Since food is "input" and exercise or activity is "output", finding that balance between input and output is the key to weight maintenance.

The difference between someone who has an office job and someone who has a job involving physical labor could be the difference of 150 calories burned each working hour. If an average workday is eight hours, 1,200 extra calories are used each day. You can easily see how simple obesity can result from losing the delicate balance between input and output.

A slow metabolism can be kick-started in a few different ways with exercise. When you exercise with intensity, your body has to rebuild everything that you've exhausted. Your body uses calories to replenish energy resources, perform minor muscular tissue repair, re-oxygenate blood, decrease body temperature, and return ventilation and heart rate to normal. This accounts for extra calories burned following high intensity exercise. These are calories over and above the initial calories spent while doing the exercise and are directly proportional to the intensity of the exercise. This phenomenon is often referred to as *Excess Post Exercise Oxygen Consumption (EPOC)*. The number is higher in weight lifting than aerobic activity. If you were to exercise with intensity every day, your metabolism would actually increase. In other words, you would become more efficient at burning body fat through disciplined exercise.

Energy Sources: The body uses its energy sources differently. The quickest and strongest muscle contractions use sugar as an energy source. Weight lifting burns plenty of sugar or "glucose" because of the short duration and explosive nature of the exercise. Muscles do not utilize oxygen during intense weight-lifting exercises (anaerobic).

When beginning an exercise, muscles are powered almost exclusively by the immediate energy source, glucose. If exercise continues to become more intense, the body will start demanding more oxygen. If the exercise becomes too intense for regular controlled breathing, oxygen cannot be supplied through the bloodstream at the elevated demand, and the exercise goes from an "aerobic" exercise to an "*an*aerobic" exercise. During heavy weight lifting, the exercises are too demanding to supply oxygen to the muscle that is being worked. A burning sensation in the working muscle occurs when the muscle begins to fatigue. The burn is caused by "lactic acid". This acid is a by-product of glucose burned without oxygen. This is a normal and necessary chemical reaction when weight lifting. For maximum results from weight lifting, it is important to "feel the burn". Over the course of a workout, as sugar (glucose) becomes less readily available, a maximum muscle contraction becomes more difficult. Weight lifting is most efficient when sugar (glucose) is at its peak, that is, at the beginning of a workout routine.

The truth is, both sugar and fat are always feeding the muscles during aerobic activity; but their relationship is inversely proportional to each other. As glucose is used more and more in exercise, it eventually is less and less plentiful and fat plays a more active role in feeding the muscles during aerobic activity.

So, since sugar (glucose) starts strong at the beginning of exercise, fat will be used for energy in higher proportion when sugar is less available later in the same aerobic exercise session. Although fat is not metabolized for energy during weight lifting (or at least in much less proportion than sugar), it metabolizes nicely with plenty of oxygen and is a good aerobic energy source when glucose is low.

In order to perform an intense weight lifting program, sugar (glucose) availability should be at its highest level. Simply put, weight training activity done prior to aerobic activity will best utilize your body's natural sugar (glucose) storage. Also, aerobic exercise assists in the removal of lactic acid that is built-up from weight lifting by flooding the muscles with fresh oxygenated blood. This reduces the potential for ongoing muscle soreness.

Clearly, doing weight training (anaerobic exercise) first, while you have full glucose reserves, gives you the exercise results. Remember, the fact that you do any exercise, is far more important than the order of exercise. The key to speeding up the body's metabolism safely and naturally is by starting a disciplined exercise routine.

Integration: An interesting study of Canadian Mennonite children provides a little insight into the development of the epidemic of our overweight children. The study shows that a traditional way of life—that is, physical labor and physical play—may reduce chronic disease. The results of the study suggest that children who live a lifestyle somewhat representative of previous generations (Mennonite lifestyle: no television, video games, or processed foods) are leaner and stronger than children living a contemporary Canadian lifestyle. In other words, the sedentary behaviors adopted by our current lifestyles have mostly contributed to the obesity epidemic in our children.

During the agricultural age, labor was physical and play was outdoors. Yesterday's rope swing and physical games have been replaced, for the majority of adolescents, by the video game and television. The fruits and vegetables from the fields of sixty years ago are replaced with today's processed combo meals.

If neglected, exercise and a healthy diet has a high price to pay in the long run if it is not integrated into one's daily schedule, especially in our children.

Exercise should not have to be another commitment to be penciled into an already busy daily agenda. Exercise is a lifestyle change. It is looking at your life differently. Instead of seeing the day as a series of to-do activities in which exercise is just another activity, exercise should just be part of an overall healthier lifestyle.

Integrating exercise into a healthy lifestyle might mean your lunch break is thirty minutes on a treadmill and a fruit salad instead of a hamburger and fries. It might entail a run in the morning before a shower. It might be walking with a significant other at night. As you walk off the frustrations of the day with exercise, you and your spouse, friend, or exercise partner are accountable to and supportive of each other in your fitness plans. Exercise could also be integrated into what happens at your place of worship—exercise with prayer or with a study group that creatively ties wellness with devotions: faith with fitness.

Exercise is a lifestyle change that is addictive—in a good way—if it is done consistently and as a priority. Before long, you will find that all other things will fall into place. You will see that you're changing your eating habits because you become acutely aware of empty calories; and you begin to feel compassion for those who go without food. Your friends, children, and community see you; and in turn, they may become inspired by your efforts and join the cause. Expect to excite others with the healthy habits that you decided to adopt. Those who see you as a model of improved health will be strengthened by your determination and inspired to stop abusive behaviors. Your community will follow your lead and live happier and healthier lives because you decided to *care for yourself so you could better care for them.*

Create a lifestyle that allows the space and time for healthy living. Do the following, if you are able:

Climb stairs instead of using elevators
Park in the back of parking lots
Get on the floor with children
Walk everywhere you can
Bicycle more, Drive less
Dance
Turn off the television
Replace the desk chair with a Therapy Ball
Give thanks for the gift of movement
Discover exercise as a spiritual discipline

Nature: Richard Louv, author of *Last Child in the Woods,* came to disturbing conclusions in his work with adolescents. He discovered that the recent switch from outdoor (natural) play to indoor television and video games are linked directly to the trends of childhood obesity, Attention Deficit Disorder (ADD), and depression.

When it is time to vacation, consider the wilderness. The hiking trails, camps, canoeing, or other outdoor activities often create a closer connection to the Creator and your community. The many summers I took church groups to hike the Appalachian Trail created a complete experience of fellowship, devotion, physical challenges, support, and overall goodwill of a community. In addition to the physical support each member of the hiking community gives to ensure everyone gets safely over and through the rocks and creeks; the community supports each other with its use of food rations. The stronger and more able hikers carry more weight than those who cannot. Skilled individuals support the community with their knowledge of fire building, cooking, and trail safety. All are cared for as needed. Every member has a part. Every member is vital to the health and safety of the community.

The culture of the hiking community in the national parks, the Appalachian Trail, and other national trails is to "leave no trace". It is the ecological responsibility of the individual to keep the natural resources intact for the wildlife, future visitors, and the larger global community. "Leave no trace" can be adapted to our everyday life and our interaction with our God-given resources. Being a good steward of our land will leave these resources for future generations.

Nature offers simplicity. When you are hiking, it is just you and the sounds of creation. Without cell phones, computers, televisions, and even automobiles; life is more simply lived and with greater clarity. Through nature, it is easier to get back in touch with our community, ourselves, and God. Our relationship with our Creator is too often overshadowed by our "stuff". Get out into the woods, explore God's playground, and feel how easy it is to reconnect. Rediscover just how little we actually need to live fully. Everything needed to sustain life for days on end comes from a thirty-five-pound pack, a good pair of boots, community support, and fresh streams along the footpath.

> *I went to the woods because I wished to live deliberately, to front only the essential facts of life, and see if I could learn what it had to teach, and not, when I come to die, discover that I had not lived.*
> —*Henry David Thoreau*

When I think of being out in the elements, I am always reminded of the story of Elijah in the Old Testament. Elijah was a prophet who ran away to the mountains and away from the pressures and dangers of the world. Specifically, he was fleeing from the evil King Ahab and his Queen Jezebel in fear of his life. God told him to stand at the opening of a cave in the mountains and wait for God to "pass by". As Elijah stood at the mouth of the cave, there was an earthquake, but God was not in it. A tremendous wind blew through, like a hurricane with enough wind to smash rocks, but God wasn't in that. Then a fire appeared, but God wasn't in that either. All of this chaos was followed by silence . . . and God was there. God spoke in a 'still small voice' to Elijah. Elijah listened and understood (1 Kings 19:1-18).

When you reach the top of a mountain that you spent the last hour hiking up, you might not hear birds, insects, wind, or any sound at all at first. It is then God speaks. By removing all the distractions and listening to the silence, you will find yourself in communion with the Creator. On the mountain, in the woods, or on the ocean when the noise is gone; God's voice is heard clearly in the stillness.

Worship: Our very worship experience could be influenced for the better with exercise. Attending a worship service of a different religion can be a "physical" awakening experience. While I was in seminary, I went to a Muslim Mosque. The Imam (the Muslim congregation's worship leader) was in his early seventies; I was in my mid-thirties. The service was approximately thirty minutes long. We assumed the multi-point positions always facing toward Mecca, the most holy place for Muslims. As you might have already seen, the positions were a series of bows, kneels, squats, reaches, and prayer stretches. This was done a total of seven times during the thirty minutes. By the end of the half hour, I found myself fatigued just by this prayer practice. It is one of the core beliefs of the Islamic religion that all Muslims pray this way five times every day. The Imam outdid me physically that day, even though he was twice my age. He was fit for the very physical worship that all Muslims do everyday, five times. As I prayed to Jesus throughout the service, I could not help but notice the slight pains I felt in my knees and back and the sweat that was dripping from my forehead. However, I sensed my Muslim brothers were not focused on the pain, only on God.

In a Buddhist temple, I sat facing the temple worship leader who was in her early sixties. Like the Imam at the Mosque, she was almost twice my age. After twenty minutes in a cross-legged position on the floor, my knees, hips, and back hurt enough to interrupt my deep meditation on Christ. At the end of meditation, I noticed our worship leader jumped up from a cross-legged position; while the rest of us western Christian seminary students, not conditioned for this physical challenge in their typical worship experience, slowly stood with discomfort.

Worship at a Hindu temple combined yoga meditation and positioning throughout the entire worship. We, who were unaccustomed to this style of worship, had the hardest time with pain and concentration because of our personal deconditioned state.

Quite possibly, engaging the physical body in prayer, meditation, and worship, as most world religions do, will improve physical fitness and deepen our ability to focus on God. The Bible speaks of various positions of prayer:

1. **Standing** (Mark 11:25)
2. **Lifting hands** (Timothy 2:8)
3. **Sitting** (2 Samuel 7:18)
4. **Looking upward** (John 17:1)
5. **Bowing down** (Exodus 34:8)
6. **Placing head between the knees** (1 Kings 18:42)
7. **Kneeling** (Luke 22:41, Acts 7:60, 9:40, 20:36, 21:5; Ephesians 3:14; 2 Chronicles 6:13; Daniel 6:10)
8. **Prostrate to the Lord** (Matthew 26:39, Mark 14:35).

Various positions of prayer might allow us to experience and enhance a deeper level of meditation by fully engaging our physical bodies with the art of meditation and prayer as the ancients did. A deconditioned body tends to focus on aches, pains, restlessness, and fatigue. It has more difficulty reaching deeper levels of communion with God. Healthy eating and exercise might even assist our time with God by deepening our ability to meditate and pray without those aches, pains, restlessness, and fatigue that a deconditioned body causes.

Discipleship: If fitness is your only goal, you may be disappointed since studies show that 50 percent of the time you will fail to achieve within three to six months. Permanent weight loss will fall short by any method other than proper diet and exercise. Therefore, you need motivation that will stay with you for life. Fitness, injury prevention, and good health practices work together to improve your ability to faithfully care for others. There is a great irony in it all. The things we worry so much about, and the things we think are so important—like amassing wealth—carry little weight at the end of the journey. The only thing that consistently matters in the end is love—the love one gave and the love one felt, and the difference they made for the better. Love provides the discipline that keeps us in healthy habits of diet and exercise long after the motivation of "aesthetics" (or how we look) is gone. Because of our healthy changes, we can bring life to those who otherwise would starve. We practice *The Golden Rule*.

Summary of Exercise Benefits: Regular exercise slows the natural aging process. Daily exercise will:

1. Reverse osteoporosis
2. Reverse muscle atrophy or shrinking (sarcopenia)
3. Slow formation of arthritis
4. Decrease hypertension
5. Decrease obesity
6. Improve posture
7. Improve immune system
8. Improve short-term memory
9. Increase cardiovascular output
10. Lower the risk of many cancers
11. Lower risk of diabetes
12. Regulate sleep patterns
13. Improve muscle balance and coordination
14. Decrease depression, anxiety, and stress
15. Improve self-image
16. Protect against Alzheimer's disease and dementia
17. Reduce healthcare costs
18. Increases metabolism
19. Helps reconnect mind, body, and spirit

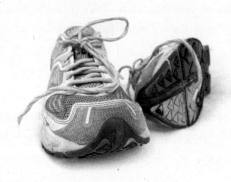

FAITH

Our efforts made towards personal fitness can become a true spiritual discipline, an expression of gratitude, and thanksgiving for all of life. When we learn to care for ourselves to better care for others, we simplify and intensify our quest towards personal fitness.

I offer you a true story that was first written in the introduction of *Wellplanet (2010)*. It is the story of Agnes. Agnes was one completely forgotten by an unfortunate combination of dementia, old age, and poverty. Yet, even in her deep despair of pitiful brokenness, God's grace went deeper still to comfort Agnes.

All caregivers who work with senior adults know that each patient is a professor with a lesson to teach. One simply needs eyes that are open and ears to hear. Here is Agnes' story.

"Help me! I'm in the valley...help!" You learn to ignore cries like these when you have been working in the nursing home settings for almost two full decades.

Walking the halls, carrying a walker, a safety belt, a clip board, and a pair of crutches under my arm, I was pacing myself to visit ten elderly patients that day. I was doing quite well with my steady pace.

"Help me! I'm in the valley...help!"

I heard the voice again off in the distance. It was a desperate woman's cry. But again, this was not a bit unusual. The moans and shouts you hear like this behind closed doors of our senior facility were normal. In fact, I had come to believe I was immune to them. I've been told you can get used to anything if you do it long enough.

I had finished with rooms 4C and 6C and started heading to the A wing. I was still early, I was budgeting my time wisely that morning. I had almost walked by when I heard the cry once more.

"Help me! I'm in the valley...help!"

I was already making good time and I debated: "do I push on and go home early or do I take the time to explore the voice behind the door?" I wasn't sure what I would find. A thought occurred to me that maybe the woman did indeed slide off her bed and was wedged between her bed and the wall. She would quite literally be "in the valley", under just such a scenario. I had an obligation to respond to her rescue; so I took a moment to explore.

I put down the walker I was carrying, untangled the crutches from my safety belt, laid down my clipboard, and slowly eased the door open to the woman's room.

I saw her as I entered the room, a tiny frail African American woman sitting in a wheelchair built for someone twice the size of her 80 pound frame. She was well over ninety, blind, wasted muscles, stooped over with osteoporosis, and confined to her wheelchair. I could tell she was very scared—so much so, she had tears streaming from the corners of her glazed-over eyes. There was no telling how long she had been crying.

"Good morning. Can I help you?"

Hearing my voice, she reached out her crippled hands into the empty space where she thought I would be, sensing that I was now in the room.

"Help me! I'm in the valley...help!" The genuine pain and anguish that this elderly woman was exhibiting left me with a feeling of hopelessness. *"Help me! I'm in the valley...help! Please help me! I'm in the valley!"*

I could not mistake what she meant. It doesn't take a religious degree to know of what "valley" she was speaking about. Any young person who spent a few months in Sunday school, maybe a week at Bible camp, or attended a funeral knows the reference to Psalms 23 – "the valley of the shadow of death". In this poor woman's advanced dementia, her head was telling her that she was quite literally walking through the valley of the shadow of death! Frightened for her life, she desperately cried out for help.

My heart broke but what could I do? She had dementia; she wouldn't understand any reasoning, would she?

I glanced at the woman's name bracelet. "Agnes", I said calmly to her. "Do you remember the rest of that psalm?" I took her trembling hand and leaned close to her ear. "Even though I walk through the valley of the shadow of death, I will fear no evil, for thou art with me, thy. . . ."

Before I finished that line she had joined me in perfect unison: "…Thy rod and thy staff, they comfort me…Thou preparist a table before me in the presence of my enemies!"

In the blink of an eye, I was a witness to a complete metamorphosis of emotions. Her tears of anguish changed into tears of joy in that instant. Her face shifted from pain to blessed assurance.

"I will fear no evil!" she continued. "I will fear no evil! Praise Jesus! He is with me! I am still in the valley but I am no longer afraid, praise Jesus! I am not afraid, no valley (will) scare me! I am no longer afraid!"

I slowly guided her hand back to the armrest of the wheelchair. I bid her a quiet goodbye; but she was oblivious to my presence, completely unaware that I was leaving the room. With tears of joy and a huge toothless smile, she was praising her Jesus for walking with her through the *valley of the shadow of death* with no fear, only joy.

As the morning progressed, I passed the door again. I could hear soft comforted noises coming from her room. Just a little later, I could hear hymns of praise as I passed by. She had a comforted heart. Completely confused, but comforted all the same. Agnes had a mind that was beyond proper function, but a fully comforted heart.

The thoughts of her savior lasted all day. I can only assume she was comforted as long as she remembered her Jesus; but when dementia got the best of what was left of her memories, she returned back to the valley alone, trying desperately to find comfort when she could not remember her way.

Maybe it was the dementia, maybe it was just Agnes hoping for comfort; but at that moment, "faith" literally was the difference between life and death. In spite of compounded earthly hardships of old age—living in a nursing home, dementia, blindness, pain, and anxiety— Agnes still experienced holy peace and holy comfort. She had a hopeful 'way' to see life, with no more fear.

Stepping *inside* our own religious practices is to not simply *hope* in God, but stepping inside our religion is to release anxiety and *trust* God completely.

Like The Golden Rule, this new *way* of trusting God, trusting *outside* ourselves, is encouraged by Jesus and all the great spiritual teachers. It is this great way of trusting God that transcends all religious ritual and practice. It is God drawing us to Him, regardless of what name we learned to call Him. This *great way* of trust can only happen when the road that leads to Him is clear of our own anxieties, egos, and prejudices. These things clutter debris across the path that journeys to God. Since God is love, love is the *great way to God*. We need not to fear the details of religion and proper practice we have learned from our childhood lessons. We need to only fear forgetting that the single purpose to our religion is God leading us to love Him. Love is what matters, for this was Jesus' message, and in this message we can trust completely. Love is the *great way* that transcends our religious framework we have learned. Buddha said "If I had even a slight awareness and practiced the *Great Way* what I would fear would be deviating from it".

Theology, in the classic sense, is to study God; to learn about God. *Religion* is a systematic set of beliefs and practices based on a common theology. Christianity, like Buddhism, Islam, Hinduism, and Judaism, is a religion in the practical sense. Yet, a set of beliefs based on a common theology is not what gave Agnes comfort. Agnes most likely learned *about* God through the childhood faith handed down from her parent's church. But at some point, faith in God became personal, very personal. She had *met* God in Jesus. That is what gave her peace—the person of Jesus, who walked in the valley with her. She *felt* his love.

You can see that for Agnes, following God meant to step outside the knowing *about* God, and into *knowing* Him personally. Religion for Agnes is not merely adhering to a systemic set of common practices, but it is trusting His 'way'. She moved from extreme fear to a place of peace and comfort because of a faith that assured her she was with Jesus in a frightening circumstance.

Was this a real encounter? I do not know how to answer that. To her it is as real as the pages you are reading. To a psychologist or sociologist studying human behaviors, it might be that she had made manifest what she had hoped for in her 90 plus years of life. Either way, God does work in mysterious ways.

Was this a real encounter? It is as difficult as answering the question "is love real?" It is a question one cannot answer without experiencing it first.

So it goes with the elderly. Comfort does not always come easily. As we reach the final chapter of our lives, we prepare for the final exam, so to speak. With advancing physical infirmness, life has an ironic *way* of allotting an opportunity to grow in *spirit* as the physical body declines. Hundreds of elderly, with whom I have had the pleasure to spend their final days, come to an end of their journey and most everyone echoed the same conclusion: God offered a way out of the suffering.

Problems and challenges will always be part of the human experience. *But, is it really possible to stop fighting the darkness of our fears simply by ushering in the light of God's love, as Agnes did?*

We discover the importance of our faith in times of great tribulation. But if we allow God's Spirit to walk with us through every arena of life-even the "grit" of our daily lives, our perceptions of life's difficulties change. Like the profound story of Agnes, we no longer try to be brave-we are brave; we no longer try to be joyful-we are joyful; we don't need to try to be patient-we simply are patient. These are the manifestations of trusting our higher power; it does not come from our making or doing, it simply is. We think and live a new way.

But just how can this *spiritual* trust affect our *temporal* lives and relationships? The peace of mind is the *fruit* produced by entrusting our lives to God and letting go of our need to *control* our lives. We dissolve our ego, we no longer amass hurts and disappointments, and we travel lighter-physically and emotionally. Essentially, we stop fighting the evils of darkness, and allow in the light of God's love and guidance. When we do this, we live a new way and everything changes. Gluttony, apathy, fear and frustration have no more shadows to hide behind anymore, and this is the crux of a relationship that we nurture with our God.

Without realizing our inherent hunger for our source of life, the "God-shaped holes" in our hearts remain unfilled. We turn away from our God, who is love; and in time, we manifest even more pain and emptiness, and walk through our valley, alone. Unfortunately, pangs of emptiness, loneliness, and lack of fulfillment lead some individuals to numb the pain with harmful substances like alcohol, drugs, and even comfort foods. These substitutions for love ultimately lead us away from personal health.

Like Agnes, we begin our journey to health and happiness by learning to trust the Creator. When we surrender fighting the evils of darkness and allow God's light to shine in; then we begin to discover the fullness of peace, comfort, and understanding that will lead to a healthy mind, body, and spirit.

Mind, Body, and Spirit Connection

An interesting study was done with rabbits at Ohio State University in the 1970's. In the study, many caged rabbits were being fed incredibly toxic, high-cholesterol diets in order to study the effects of poor diet and blocked arteries. All the rabbit groups that were in cages showed almost the exact same results of heart disease after a period of time. All the same, except one group of rabbits. That particular group of rabbits had 60% less symptoms of heart disease than all the other rabbits. Nothing in the study showed a difference in the variables. Each group got exactly the same fatty foods and water. There physiology should not show any difference between the groups. All variables were the same.

The scientists were puzzled. No variables were different, yet one particular group of rabbits experienced 60% better health than all the others. Finally one day, an observation was made by a professor when he witnessed the student who was in charge of that one particular group of rabbits. It appears that this particular student was a bleeding heart, a real lover of animals. When she would feed and clean the cages, unlike all the other students who cared for all the other cages, this student took a long time with each rabbit. She delighted in petting them and sharing her love with each one.

This was the only difference. The rabbits felt no fear about their handling; they were calm and worry free. They felt loved. As far as they knew, the giant hand that lifted them from the cage and fed them was the loving hand of God. That alone reduced their heart disease 60% over the others who were typical scared rabbits. Trusting a loving God released the anxiety and worry in the rabbits and created the difference. The study was repeated and results were the same. Love exponentially increased the health of the rabbits by reducing anxiety and stress.

> *Do not worry about your life...look at the birds of the air, they will not reap or sow or store away in barns, yet your heavenly father provides for them, how much more will He do for you?*
> *-Jesus (Matthew 6:25-26)*

Prayer & mediation, exercise, and drugs like cocaine, affect the brain similarly. As mentioned in the last chapter, both exercise and certain addictive drugs tell the brain through a neurotransmitter "dopamine" that the body needs more. In other words the body starts to crave more of what it had received whether it is alcohol, cocaine, or exercise. Dopamine that is released in the brain begins the process of addiction. Exercise, like cocaine or alcohol, stimulates the brain to crave what it just received. With ongoing exercise, the body learns to crave this exercise. Over time the healthy routine of exercise becomes an ongoing positive response to the body craving exercise. It becomes a healthy addiction.

Rats in cages with running wheels show less interest in drug stimulants than rats without exercise options. The bottom line is this: the more you exercise over time, the more you will want to exercise. Healthy habits are formed for life with ongoing exercise.

Meditation and prayer stimulate the brain much like exercise. Specifically, meditation stimulates the frontal lobes of the brain. This is the area of the brain where the highest levels of concentration occurs.

Monks, of both Christian and Buddhist traditions who have trained their entire lives in the practices of meditation and contemplative prayer, have learned to master this thought pattern in the brain. When the monks pray, the neurotransmitter activity in the "parietal lobes" decrease, while activity in the "frontal lobes" greatly increase. In other words, the *chatter* stops and one thought becomes razor sharp. That thought is of God.

The monks, who focus on God, learn to think only of Him during meditation and contemplative prayer. The inward focus on God can be clearly seen in clinical trials with these trained monks. The clinical trials explain the outward manifestation of peace these monks have in their everyday lives.

Trained monks who practice and master meditation possess a "peace that passes all understanding"; a sharp reduction of stress levels over the general public. These monks exhibit exponential reductions in blood pressure, anxiety, chronic pain, irritable bowel syndrome, hyperactivity, and other ailments that are linked directly to stress.

Caring for ourselves physically, mentally, and spiritually can start by simply learning to meditate on God, while beginning and sustaining an ongoing exercise routine.

If we learn to exercise while practicing meditation, we learn to shut off the chatter while receiving the health benefits of exercise. Eventually, one finds physical health while finding that inner-peace.

Exercise and prayer are the beginning steps to caring for ourselves physically, mentally, and spiritually.

People of the *Way*

"The Way" was one of the original terms that defined the beginnings of the Christian movement through the first century. The *Way* was used to describe this 'new way' of living and treating each other. We learn all about the people of the *Way* throughout the book of Acts and Paul's letters in the New Testament. As with any new community, this first-century group of believers had trials and struggles. The most revealing piece of the puzzle we get of those original people of the *Way* was that they didn't function as individuals, but each functioned as a valuable member of the larger community. In other words, when the individual was in good fortune, the whole community benefited; and when the individual was in need, the entire community was there to respond by sharing.

> *Now the whole group of those who believed were of one heart and soul, and no one claimed private ownership of any possessions, but everything they owned was held in common (Acts 4:32).*

This was the original snapshot of the Christian movement—collective good will for all. Being of one heart and soul, sprung the original community of the new *Way* to collectively bring the message of God's revelation of love through Jesus to a global religion over the following centuries. It was the alternative *way* to live, not in despair, but in mutual respect and love for each other. This *way* of caring for each other was alien to the people of the Roman Empire; it was noticed and found to be attractive to some . . . and then more. This *Way* added numbers to their mission every day. The original community grew dramatically, without force, but with gentleness and compassion. So salvation was not just seen as a ticket to heaven, but *The Way* meant salvation from living in daily despair, alone. This *way* of compassion is the spiritual path Jesus walked. It was God's will on earth, as it is in heaven.

The religious community was represented poorly by the sword during the crusades of the Middle Ages. In fact, historically, when this original model of compassion had been neglected, the spread of Christianity had wavered. The harder one tries to force the virtues of *The Way*, the less authentic it becomes. *The Way* is the "theology of the towel" as we read in the gospel of John (Jesus washing the feet of the disciples, and then instructing them to do likewise). This is a victory that cannot be won on the battlefield. It is a victory of the heart.

The quintessential Christian symbol is the cross. It symbolizes the final victory through one laying down his life for others. Living not for the self, but for the salvation of all humanity. The crucifixion demonstrated fully the abandonment of the self for the benefit of all.

The story, "The Rabbi's Gift," introduces the abandonment of *"self"* for the benefit of all. This is the compassionate world of respect that The Golden Rule teaches. It is not the sensational story of God's spirit descending on the first believers that we read in the book of Acts. But all the same, the Holy Spirit is still present. There is no speaking in many languages, no tongues of fire, no supernatural revelation; but there is a love and respect for the community. This love and respect is the profound revelation that is powerful and simple enough to change the world. Here is the story:

> The monastery with the chapel on the hill had fallen apart; no one wished to come anymore. Just three elderly monks were left in this dilapidated old order. Once a solid chapel, now it stood in ruin, with no money to fix it and no congregation to care.
>
> The three brothers constantly blamed each other. "No one is here because of the two of you. If you weren't so mean, people might come!" the first brother would say. Another one said, "Your frustration caused our entire congregation to leave and not come back!"

And the third brother would say, "It is the two of you who caused us this problem, for you two think only of yourselves!"

On and on it went, month after month and year after year. The brothers remained frustrated with each other.

One day a rabbi came to visit his three friends at this dying chapel. The three brothers pleaded with the rabbi for advice to save the monastery. They dined together and cried together. Even the rabbi could tell that the Spirit had left his three friends, and he knew that the people who lived down in the village below the chapel had also lost the Spirit.

The rabbi left with these words, "I am so sorry I couldn't save the chapel, but I know the Messiah lives in one of you" and with that he left. What was this strange message that the rabbi left them? Could it be a code for something bigger? Could he possibly be talking about one of them? The brothers contemplated.

In the days that followed, the three brothers pondered the statement of the rabbi. "Maybe the Messiah lives in my brother. No, maybe it is me that he lives in, or maybe it is in my other brother."

As they continued to ponder the statement, something miraculous began to happen. From the thought of Christ living in the heart of one of the brothers, an extraordinary respect for all of the brothers began to grow. The glow of compassion, respect, and love began to exude from each of them; and it was both attractive and contagious. The aura began to flow down the hill and into the village. Within a short time, villagers began to wander toward the old chapel to warm up in its glow. The Spirit was in the air. Before long, the chapel became a center for a thriving community once again— thanks to the rabbi's gift.

A monastery, church, synagogue, or other religious communities start, struggle, and grow because of a disciplined compassion of its members. A faith community grows stronger proportionately to the healthy "time" they spend in fellowship and welcoming. Ironically, our nation's communities are spending less quality time with each other than previous generations. Robert Putnam, in his book *Bowling Alone*, shows a detailed trend in which most all the groups, clubs, events, or routines that used to draw us together in community have declined sharply in the last sixty years. Church attendance, PTA, league bowling, social groups, political parties, and civic clubs have all decreased in membership and participation. Along with this trend toward less group interaction and fellowship, there had been a rise in entertainment and "spectator" activities such as television, movies at home, and computer games; as well as social media like Facebook™. As we choose spectator activities over interactive face-to-face activities, we move away from the fellowship common to the generations before us. We engage with less "depth" with one another. Even though we are getting more connected via Facebook™, text messaging, and emails; social media just cannot provide the same depth that actual fellowship provides.

In a 2012 article in the Atlantic Magazine, Stephen Marche observed a startling contradiction. He wrote:

> *"Within this world of instant and absolute communication, unbounded by the limits of time and space, we suffer from unprecedented alienation. We have never been more detached from one another or lonelier."*

A "true" community lives face-to-face and social media can enhance the community's relationships; but the bonds of friendship are built by members giving their whole selves to each other being completely present, honest, and "real" with another. Fellowship is necessary for spiritual growth among people. Being real means to come to commune with all the baggage: imperfect, broken, and honest. In order to grow, one must risk this pain and vulnerability. Otherwise, a community will always remain superficial with walls carefully guarded between its members, not requiring risk among its members. No risk, no pain, no growth. Our spiritual health requires growth and interconnectedness. It is the difference between "disciplined ongoing fellowship" and occasional socializing. Sherry Turkle, in her 2011 book *Alone Together* said this: "The ties we form through the Internet are not, in the end, the ties that bind, but they are the ties that preoccupy".

Our physical and spiritual health require discipline. One must eat healthy and exercise for their physical health. Likewise, one must be disciplined in caring for others in order to foster deeper and more meaningful spiritual connections with their community members. There are no shortcuts. When we "care for ourselves to better care for others", our lives become more in line with "The Golden Rule". We can now see exercise and healthy eating foster deeper loving relationships as spiritual disciplines.

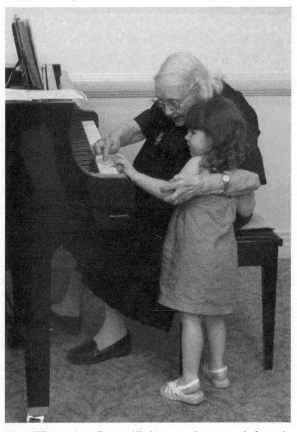

Alma (97) teaches Emma (4) how to play piano before the Village Chapel Intergenerational Church Service.

www.gulfcoastvillagechapel.com

(Photo www.dekoter.net)

The Last Chapter

Charles Dickens immortalized the character of Ebenezer Scrooge. The outlook of this character changed overnight with the help of three ghosts. The story ends with Ebenezer understanding the value of loving your neighbor. That story speaks to us so plainly; because it plays out the consequences of our free choice to be "in communion with" or "alienated from" the community around us. Unfortunately, in real life we don't get clarity from the help of three well-meaning spirits. We are given free choice to make that decision for ourselves. We are free to choose to practice The Golden Rule as all religions point towards, or we can choose not to. Likewise, we can choose to exercise and eat healthy, or chose not to. In the end, whatever choices we make, we live with the consequences.

Walter

While looking out over the snow-covered ground outside of his second story nursing home window in rural eastern Pennsylvania, Walter drifts in and out of shallow catnaps. This has been his daily routine for nearly two years, with few breaks. There were the two Christmas events when his son brought him out of the home, and the several day trips he took on the community bus. But every other day since he'd moved there included the routine of watching the seasons change out of his window.

From a distance he hears the faint sound of the golden oldies station. It is Glenn Miller. Walter is awake again and reliving the tremendous feeling of freedom when returning home from Italy after the war ended. Wide awake, Walter is pleased and content as he reflects on his life.

His body was different then. He has a picture of himself and a few army buddies on his wall. One soldier in the photo never came home. While sailing on two very small ships, they were ambushed by German soldiers. The rear vessel went down with no survivors. Walter was in the lead boat, and the eight men on his boat survived. In the picture, the soldiers are dressed in their green army fatigues, which are a non-distinct dark shade in the faded black-and-white picture. The photo shows his posture is upright, his frame is heavily muscled with straight legs, and his shoulders do not slump forward as they do now. He stands with perfect posture sixty years earlier.

After the war, Walter had returned to work as an accountant. His occupation required long hours of sitting. His diet during his years was ethnically laced with Pennsylvania Dutch pan-fried potatoes and large portions of meat. He admitted that only on rare occasions did he eat seasonal vegetables or fruit. He had no set exercise patterns or routines all his adult life.

Nearing ninety, Walter's physical condition includes a compression fracture of a vertebra between his shoulder blades, an old hip fracture with a total hip replacement, shoulder problems, and neck pain with prior surgery for arthritis. Arthritis has conquered the knees as well. In addition to this, Walter is unable to stand erect because of arthritis and muscle weakness. Unfortunately, this keeps him in a wheelchair.

If a body is limited to a sitting position, endurance is greatly compromised. Walter's legs are contracted. Because of being in a constant sitting position for more than two years, he is unable to stand or extend his knees completely straight. His loss of flexibility causes pain in his back and legs when he occasionally attempts to rise from his chair. Prolonged sitting also effects the heart, lungs, and circulation; and of course, without the freedom of movement, obesity becomes a problem.

When an adult body does not get exercised, it will lose its strength and muscle size (sarcopenia). A human can lose up to one-percent of his or her muscle size every year after the age of twenty-five. It is easy to see how this can begin to lead to an early disability by robbing the leg muscles of the strength to carry the weight of the body or even lift it from a chair.

Looking at Walter's shoulders, he has what is called a rotator cuff tear. Unfortunately, he has it in both shoulders. The rotator cuff is four small muscles that hold the shoulder joint in place while the big muscles of the shoulder move the arm. The muscles of the rotator cuff are thin to begin with and, as we age due to the effects of sarcopenia, they get thinner and weaker. One day, when a senior citizen reaches for something heavy or catches himself from a fall, the rotator cuff tears. Unfortunately, with a tear, the arm does not work well. Reaching overhead becomes nearly impossible. Lifting heavy objects also becomes very difficult. Even though it is a small group of muscles, they can cause a great deal of disability. Surgery and a lengthy rehabilitation can correct the problem a great majority of the time. More than four million Americans like Walter seek surgeons for shoulder problems of this type each year.

In Walter's case, his spinal and hip fractures were a direct result of osteoporosis. Osteoporosis is loss of bone mineral in which the remainder of the bone is brittle and easily fractured. Posture changes in older adults are usually caused by the combined effects of osteoporosis, sarcopenia, and gravity. Endurance declines with lack of exercise and the body becomes quickly disabled—unable to move a distance without becoming short of breath. Obesity becomes a factor when activity is diminished simply because movement burns calories. Flexibility is lost when a muscle or joint is not used or exercised through its normal available range of motion.

All of Walter's physical problems have been a result of inactivity and poor diet since returning home from WWII. So Walter sits, remembering the days of youth when he did not need a wheelchair. But Walter is a deep and compassionate thinker. He subconsciously sees a wartime event that plays over and over in his head. It is a time when he and another army private found two German soldiers. The mission was to walk them at gunpoint many miles to where the base was so they could be kept as prisoners. Evening was coming and the sky was darkening. Walter insisted that they carry through the mission while the other private, in fear for his life, felt they needed to dispose of the prisoners.

After walking several more miles along a river, evening came and the paranoia increased for both of these American heroes. The men were forced to be guided by only the sound of the rushing water, because sight was no longer useful. Without further consultation, Walter's companion knelt the two prisoners next to the river and shot both of them, each with a single bullet in the back of their heads. Years later, Walter would say through misty eyes, "It was wartime. That private wasn't thinking rationally like he would at other times".

This scenario replayed in Walter's head many times since 1944. When I first saw him staring out the window, I would think, "what can he possibly be thinking about?". But once I got to know him, I understood that Walter was searching for ways that he could have intervened to save the lives of the two German human beings. For you see, Walter subscribes to the Golden Rule. He is gentle and compassionate. He says prayers not just at night, but many times throughout the day. He is a real treat for the nursing home staff. Oftentimes, he is chosen by the employees of the home as someone to celebrate. Administrators like to introduce him to potential residents' families because of his pleasant demeanor and the sincere, playful banter that he is able to engage others in. Walter is contented. He has a strong sense of self and purpose. Unfortunately, someone did not let him know thirty years ago that if he were to exercise and balance his diet better; he probably would not need the wheelchair now and most likely would be functional and ambulatory at one hundred years old.

At this stage of Walter's life, to walk again, to stand up straight, and to have his fragile body keep up with his nimble mind would be wonderful. Walter is thankful for his nimble mind. In fact, he is thankful for many things. His grateful attitude is what makes him contented and loving toward others. It is why family, friends, and nursing home employees visit him daily. Even with his frailties and painful memories, he allows love for others to direct his conduct. In fact, the elder adults who understand the power of love are the ones who are most likely to be contented with their lives at this stage. It is the love they possess that overshadows the discomfort of memories past and the pain of feeble bodies—bodies that were once sturdy and capable.

Reflecting on what is important throughout the marathon of life, most senior adults agree that love is the ultimate prize and the reason to keep running. It may not always be clear during the race, but it is crystal clear at the finish.

The seniors in our lives give us a window looking into our own futures. So many senior adults, like Walter, embrace love as a primary motive in life. Again and again, stories echo the significance of a fulfilled life when love is the catalyst. During their final years, many seniors feel a life of fulfillment with love. Sadly, those who lived a self-serving existence reflect something very different in their final years. Either way, we can learn from what they have to teach us.

Mary

Mary was frustrated. She was in her late seventies, focused on her own needs, and incensed at the fact that her disabilities kept her from her activities. The activities are why she moved to Florida years ago. Mary had a niece who helped her with daily activities, but she had no husband or children. The niece visited her out of family obligation. Mary had a sister, but they were not close. She had no real relationships and no friends. Everyone avoided her—except out of duty. She was intolerant of the staff. Mary had no other visitors, but her roommate did. During one of those visits, a curtain opened. On the other side of the curtain was a cute six-year-old girl who was spending time with her grandma in the next bed. Mary pointed to the girl and said "put me in another room. I hate kids, and I don't want anything to do with them". The family visiting will never forget those words, especially the little girl. It was obvious to see that anyone entering Mary's life was soon rejected in the wake of her massive frustration and anger. She affected everyone by her mere presence. As a highly educated former athlete, she had all the advantages growing up; but she appeared to be incapable of love or even establishing a lasting friendship. Her life was isolated, and she lived in a self-serving manner. This preoccupation with herself intensified as she grew older. She had a nimble mind, but chose to focus on her feeble body with frustration.

Like Walter, Mary had shoulder, knee, hip, and neck problems. She was affected by osteoporosis, sarcopenia, and postural difficulties. She had problems with obesity and, as with Walter, the effects of the ailments could have been reduced or reversed if Mary had disciplined herself with proper exercise and healthy habits.

Unfortunately, Mary was unable to find peace. There was no love in her life. She experienced severe depression and harbored resentment toward all others who did not have her disabilities.

Eula

Eula's funeral was a reflection of how she lived her life. As I climbed the steps of the pulpit to speak on the family's behalf, I looked out over the sea of friends and family who in one way or another had been touched by this ninety-seven-year-old woman. The old country church was full. It hadn't been this full since Easter Sunday service over nine months earlier. How could a lady of almost a century create such a following?

I remembered just a year before when I went to church with Eula and my three-year-old daughter. The pastor was talking about the resurrection, and my daughter was watching Eula. The two were sharing a moment—a human moment. A toy meant for a three year old was the magnet that brought these two together. Ninety-three years between them, both smiling and laughing as if there was nothing going on around them. It was that moment that made me remember what the magic was that attracted everyone to this contented senior. The sermon was preached from the pulpit at the front of the church, but the gospel lesson was being played out right next to me. *Practice the Golden Rule.* It's as easy as that. Eula's life was lived with both discipline and enthusiasm. She experienced God's love through everyone, young and old, who crossed her path. Her community was vast. The hundreds of people present at her funeral felt that same connection to her that my young daughter and I did just one year before.

Abner

By the time you read this, my grandfather will have died; but during the time of this writing, he lived with me. My grandfather became a resident of my personal home in his ninety-third year. His mind was still good. He could remember most of the things he had done, and the things he had left undone. While I wrote, he lay in the hospital bed that my family had set up for him in our living room. He no longer had the ability to do anything on his own, but he did reflect.

My grandfather, Pappy, was a strong man. He was a man who moved furniture for a living. Pappy retired at age sixty-five and decided to quit the physical life. Like many of his generation, retirement meant: staying at home, watching television, eating meals out, attending church and church picnics, and very little else. Pappy lived a physical life, but then he stopped. Almost thirty years later, he was unable to function independently. Arthritis had crippled his knees and hips. Sarcopenia had weakened his limbs and affected his ability to stand or pull himself to a standing position. His heart weakened, and he gained body fat from inactivity and a poor diet.

He had started to show signs of swelling in his legs from the weakened heart, skin discoloration from poor circulation, and chronic fatigue which left him sleeping the better part of the day. He was lucky to have lived as long as he did. Ninety-three is a ripe old age by any standard. Unfortunately, he had become prematurely disabled due to the accumulative affects of his inactivity and poor nutritional choices. Chances are that he could have been disability-free even in his one-hundredth year if he had been disciplined with healthy habits and exercise following his retirement.

His last days were full of wonderful memories of days gone by. His stories were rich and focused on those simpler times in which he was fully alive, serving his family on the farm with his eleven brothers and sisters before he married and moved to the city. Fond memories of his church and his civic club were among his shared stories. His peace came from the Scriptures. Until just a few weeks before the time of this writing, he was able to open his Bible on his own. Now he is unable, and I became his reader. The following was one of his favorites:

> For I am convinced that neither death, nor life, nor angels, nor rulers, nor things present, nor things to come, nor powers, nor height, nor depth, nor anything else in all creation, will be able to separate us from the love of God in Christ Jesus our Lord. — Romans 8:38-39

In the end, it was his reflection of the promise of God's love that gave him comfort. Without the love he felt, life in the end would have not made sense at all. In fact, it would have all been a tragic mistake, a pitiful existence, a selfish act of meaningless events. But, as for so many contented elderly, love built the bridge between his struggles and his understanding. Love was the catalyst for his meaningful existence. Abner's life will end content in the promise, the promise of a God who loves and provides for him; and soon, a God who will welcome him home. This is exactly like the thousands of other seniors I have had the privilage to work with over the many years of physical therapy; as well as, those that I offered pastoral care to as they slipped from this world into the next.

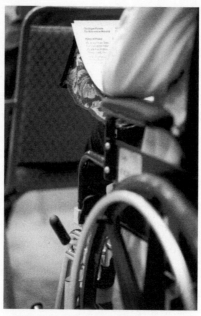

(Photo www.MelindaHawkins.com)

God is Love

"Blessed are the pure in heart, for they will see God" (Matthew 5:8). Once this is understood and once a life is lived with a pure heart full of mercy and compassion and not just concern for its own existence; life becomes meaningful, regardless of the physical limitations. Those seniors who have lived lives of only self-concern come to the end of life with an increased tendency toward frustration and depression.

Dr. Harold G. Koenig, of Duke University's *Center for the Study of Religion, Spirituality and Health* determined the following: People with strong religious faith are less likely to suffer depression from stressful life events; and if they do, they are more likely to recover from depression than those who are less religious.

Those who spend a lifetime "sowing" the seeds of love for others will reap a harvest that is bountiful in the end. Their final chapter becomes a joyful reflection of the contented life that was lived. But, when a life is spent in a self-indulgent manner no matter what the monetary or political gains; without love, in the end their harvest was pitifully scarce.

As George Bernard Shaw put it:

"This is the true joy in life—that being used for a purpose recognized by yourself as a mighty one. That being a force of nature, instead of a feverish, selfish little clod of ailments and grievances complaining that the world will not devote itself to making you happy. I am of the opinion that my life belongs to the whole community and as long as I live it is my privilege to do for it whatever I can. I want to be thoroughly used up when I die. For the harder I work the more I live. I rejoice in life for its own sake. Life is no brief candle to me. It's a sort of splendid torch which I've got to hold up for the moment and I want to make it burn as brightly as possible before handing it on to future generations."

Viktor Frankl, author of *Man's Search for Meaning*, wrote this while in his third year as a prisoner in a German Concentration camp: "love is the ultimate and the highest goal to which man can aspire".

Love reduces their emotional pain. Love is our safety net, God's shoulder to cry on. Without love, individuals who face atrocities like Auschwitz, would be forced to contemplate all of life's terrible tragedies alone. If *love is the ultimate and the highest goal to which man can aspire,* then our personal well-being depends deeply on our capacity to love. In fact, the atrocities we face due to the negligence of our neighbor can teach us the monumental importance of disciplining ourselves in practicing to love our neighbor. Past pains can lead us to mindfully practice the Golden Rule. Our negative experiences can enhance our ability to concern ourselves with the loving treatment of our neighbor.

When a child touches a hot stove, pain is felt and the child, in his limited knowledge, labels heat as bad or evil. Only through further observation and experience does he realize that heat provides warmth and comfort in the cold, and hot water for cleaning and cooking food. Eventually, the child learns that heat brings life. The old paradigm or belief that heat is evil is dropped in favor of the new understanding that heat is good and necessary.

When a child has a painful experience, she interprets the incident as best she can, and builds a belief around that experience. She might even experience God as evil or indifferent toward her because of a situation that happens. The child concludes: "I must have deserved what I got because God did not come to my rescue in my time of need" or "God just doesn't love me".

Some adults never grew spiritually, due to the limited 'bad' they have experienced in life. They stay wounded. Like the old understanding of heat, the old limited belief of a vengeful God may take new insights to correct this thinking.

The faith community provides such positive life experiences and new insights to the wounded.

"God is love" (1 John 4:16). Without believing this, we cannot understand the harmony of our co-existence with nature, with ourselves, and with each other. If one comes to believe in God's loving nature, one can begin to grasp God's provisions for us through food and exercise.

For the affluent, this much is certain: there will always be plenty of new diets, appetite suppressants, medicines, and fitness devices to fight the battle of overabundance leading to obesity and poor health. Although these items can be helpful, weight-loss attempts not understood beyond our own self-interests, traditionally fail in due time. Old habits override the best intentions of any individual. But, our issue of overabundance leading to obesity and poor health is only half of the global problem. Understanding the scarce resources of our brothers and sisters will complete our global picture and enrich our perspective.

Now, we are ready to talk about a lifetime of wellness and purpose through healthy eating and exercising. From here on, weight loss and fitness are not goals in themselves that are motivated by the scale and the mirror; but instead, proper diet and exercise can add to the length and depth of each of our lives. Great health can only enhance our ability to practice *The Golden Rule*. Wellness now has a much greater goal. The goal is not fleeting or temporary; it is for life. Our health is not just for us, but for others as well. The entire global community benefits from our food choices and our healthy habits.

It boils down to these three points that you read in the introduction:

1. **Food:** *Everything we need for sustaining health and wellness has been provided for us through nature since the beginning. If not true, life would not be. Today's health crisis is not the fault of the individual, but is a manifestation of our community forgetting our blessings of real, whole, natural foods, and simple life-giving fresh water.*

2. **Exercise:** *Unlike anything we create by hand, like a car or a refrigerator which starts to breakdown when used, the body improves in every way with moderate to heavy use. Exercise is a magic pill, a fountain of youth, an anti-depressant. The body is improved in every way possible, naturally with exercise. The Creator intended for us to move and move a lot for optimum health by design.*

3. **Faith:** *Our efforts made towards personal fitness can become a true spiritual discipline, an expression of gratitude and thanksgiving for all of life. When we 'care for ourselves to better care for others', we simplify and intensify our quest towards personal fitness.*

In faith, we die to the old us and are each created in a new *"Way"*. Our poor health and destructive habits can be given up and our lives can be made new. As new creations, we have ears to hear. This opens the door to answer the health problems for both of the global extremes of overabundance and scarcity. When we are disciplined with our overabundance while concerning ourselves with the poor, a redistribution of resources occurs throughout the global community. We eat smarter. We purchase foods more carefully. We are concerned with the treatment of our natural resources. We support local farmers. We concern ourselves with ending poverty. We stay disciplined in exercise. We avoid unhealthy habits. We become better stewards of our bodies. Every dollar spent, every action taken, and yes, even every meal eaten, ultimately works for or against the health of every person in our global community as well as the global resources we all have in common. We practice *The Golden Rule* by loving our neighbor as ourselves. In this new understanding, this new paradigm shift; wellness is no longer self-centered, but centered on neighbor. This is compassionate wellness. Such a shift is permanent and all encompassing.

We are to care for ourselves to better care for others. We are to love one another. We practice The Golden Rule.

Conclusion: If we were to work towards eating 90% of our calories as seasonal, local, organic produce; as well as, receiving the beneficial blessings of daily exercise, we would:

1. Reverse osteoporosis
2. Reverse muscle atrophy (sarcopenia)
3. Slow formation of arthritis
4. Decrease hypertension
5. Decrease obesity
6. Improve posture
7. Improve immune system
8. Improve short-term memory
9. Increase cardiovascular output
10. Lower the risk of many cancers
11. Lower risk of diabetes
12. Regulate sleep patterns
13. Improve muscle balance and coordination
14. Decrease depression, anxiety, and stress
15. Improve self-image
16. Protect against Alzheimer's disease
17. Dependency on fossil fuels would reduce
18. Pollution would decline
19. Local small farms would be supported
20. Community Supported Agriculture (CSA)

When we learn to *care for ourselves to better care for others*, we simplify and intensify our quest towards personal fitness. This is the spiritual journey of *Faith & Fitness*.

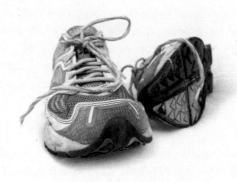

Notes

Introduction

1. Armstrong, Karen, *Twelve Steps to a Compassionate Life* (New York: Anchor Books, 2011), 3-4.

Chapter 1: Food

1. Fuhrman M.D., Joel, *Eat to Live* (New York: Time Warner, 2003).

2. Food, Field Reporter, March 20, 1939. Cited from Paradox of Plenty, 21.

3. U.S. Congressional Research Service, *"The Role of the Federal Government in Human Nutrition Research"* (Washington, D.C.: USGPO, 1976), 116. Cited from Paradox of Plenty, 74.

4. Time, Dec. 7, 1959. Cited from Paradox of Plenty, 115.

5. Nestle, Marion, *Food Politics* (Berkeley and Los Angeles: University of California Press, 2003), 11.

6. Ibid., 11.

7. Ibid., 8.

8. http://www.vegetarian-nutrition.info/nuggets/child_obesity.php.

9. New York Times, April 25, 1961. *Cited from Paradox of Plenty*, 167.

10. Nestle, Marion, Food Politics, 283. In cases like the ephedrine-containing supplements for weight loss, the FDA reported more than eight hundred cases of side-effects and twenty to thirty deaths between 1993 and 1997. Even so, in 1999, just one top selling ephedrine-containing supplement generated sales of $900 million. Finally, in 2003, the FDA recommended a ban on the sale of these products. Even with the strong warnings, they are still available and continue to be marketed.

11. Sachs, Jeffery, *The End of Poverty* (London: Penguin Books, 2006)

12. Kushner, Harold, *Living a Life That Matters* (New York: Random House, 2001), 83.

13. Robbins, J., and A. Mortifee, *In Search of Balance* (Tiburon, Calif.: H. J. Kramer, 1991), 96-97.

14. Willcox, Willcox, and Suzuki, *The Okinawa Program* (New York: Clarkson Potter/Publications).

15. Ibid., 71.

16. Buettner, Dan, *"New Wrinkles on Aging,"* National Geographic (November 2005, vol. 208), 5.

17. Levenstein, Harvey, *Paradox of Plenty: A Social History of Eating in Modern America* (Berkeley and Los Angeles: University of California Press), 66.

18. Dr. David Jenkins, Toronto, Canada, had started the work on the Glycemic Index in 1981. In many studies, white bread is used as the standard of measure at 100.

19. Nestle, Marion, *Food Politics*, vii.

20. "Gandhi". Director Richard Attenborough. With Ben Kingsley and Candice Bergen. Columbia Pictures, 1982.

21. Rolls, Barbara and Robert Barnett, *The Volumetrics: Weight-Control Plan* (New York: Harper Torch, 2003).

22. Fuhrman, 7.

23. Batmanghelidj, F., *Water for Health, for Healing, for Life* (New York: Warner Books, 2003), 32-34.

24. Thoreau, Henry David, *Walden and Other Writings* (New York: McGraw-Hill, 1988), 13.

25. O'Brien P., *"Dietary Shifts and Implications for U. S. Agriculture."* American Journal of Clinical Nutrition 1995:61 (suppl.): 1390s-1396s. Young CE, Kantor LS. "Moving Toward the Food Guide Pyramid: Implications for U. S. Agriculture." (Washington, D.C.: USDA, 1999), cited in Nestle, M. Food Politics, 363.

26. Kelly Brownell, Yale Center for Eating and Weight Disorders, cited from *SuperSize Me*, Directed by Morgan Spurlock (New York: Hart Sharp Video), 2004.

27. Brownell, K., *Food Fight* (New York: McGraw-Hill, 2004), 3.

28. Ibid., 46.

29. Tremblay, Mark S., et al. "Conquering Childhood Inactivity: Is the Answer in the Past?" Medicine Et Science in Sports Et Exercise, vol. 37, no. 7, July 2005.

30. Louv, Richard, *Last Child in the Woods: Saving Our Children from Nature Deficit Disorder* (New York: Workman Publishing, 2005).

31. Spurlock, Morgan. *Supersize Me*. Directed by Morgan Spurlock (New York: Hart Sharp Video), 2004.

32. Reyte, Elizabeth, *Garbage Land: On the Secret Trail of Trash* (New York: Little, Brown and Company, 2005), 283.

33. Hepperly, P., et al., *"Environmental, Energetic, and Economic Comparisons of Organic and Conventional Farming Systems,"* BioScience, July 2005, vol. 55, no. 7.

34. Interview with Paul Hepperly in July of 2005 at the Rodale Institute.

35. Taken from the ECHO Web site (www.echonet.org).

36. Meadows, Donella, *"Our Food, Our Future,"* Organic Gardening (www.organicgardening.com/featureprint/1,7759,s1-5-20-908,00.html).

37. Robbins, John, *May All Be Fed: Diet for a New World* (New York: William Morrow and Company, Inc., 1992), 35.

38. Ibid., 34.

39. Ibid., 35.

40. Cohen, Ben and Jerry Greenfield, *Ben & Jerry's Double Dip* (New York: Simon and Schuster, 1997). 30.

41. Levenstein, Harvey, *Paradox of Plenty: A Social History of Eating in Modern America* (Berkeley and Los Angeles: University of California Press, 2003), 145. Taken from U. S. Senate, Select Committee on Nutrition and Human Needs, Nutrition and Health 2: committee print, 94th Congress, 2nd Session, 1976, 56; New York

Times, June 6, 1963; Irene Wolgamot, "The World Food Congress," JHE 55 (August 1963), 603.

42. Robbins, 35.

43. Martinez, et al. *Local Food Systems, Concepts, Impacts, and Issues.* United States Department of Agriculture Economic Research Report, number 97, May 2010.

44. Sachs, Jeffrey D., *The End of Poverty* (London: Penguin Books, 2006), 324.

45. Ibid., 325.

46. Ibid., 326.

47. Rogers, Heather, Gone Tomorrow: The Hidden Life of Garbage (New York: New York Press, 2005).

Chapter 3: Exercise

1. Bailey, Covert, *The New Fit or Fat* (New York: Houghton-Mifflin Company, 1991), 4.

2. Edward Abbey, *Abbey's Road* (New York: Dutton, 1979).

3. Rowe, Kahn, *Successful Aging* (New York: Random House, 1998).

4. Abrams, John M.D., *Overdosed America* (New York: HarperCollins, 2005), 76.

5. In 2002, an estimated $200 billion was spent on prescription drugs in America. Worldwide, American drug companies sold about twice that amount. This number has risen approximately 300 percent between 1980 and 2000. Cited from: Angell, Marcia M.D., The Truth about the Drug Companies (New York: Random House, 2004), xxii.

6. Critser, Greg, *Generation Rx* (New York: Houghton Mifflin, 2005), 2

7. Goodpaster, Bret H., Brown, Nicholas F., *"Skeletal Muscle Lipid and Its Association with Insulin Resistance: What is the Role for Exercise?"* Exercise and Sport Sciences Reviews, American College of Sports Medicine Series, July 2005, vol. 33, no. 3.

Chapter 3: FAITH

1. Nerem, RM, Levesque, MJ, JF Cornhill *'Social Environment as a factor in diet-induced atherosclerosis'* Science June 27, 1980: Vol. 208 no. 4451 pp. 1475-1476.

2. (John 13:1-17) The foot washing was a symbolic gesture for the disciples to witness during the last night before Jesus was crucified. We are to wash the feet of others. We are to serve.

3. Battle, Michael, *"How Do We Live?"* Cited in Essentials of Christian Theology (Peabody, Mass.: Westminster John Knox Press, 2003), 291.

4. Aikman, David, *Great Souls: Six Who Changed the Century* (Nashville: Word Publishing, 1998), 122-23.

5. Ackerman, Peter and Jack Duvall, *A Force More Powerful: A Century of Nonviolent Conflict* (New York: Palgrave, 2000), 66-67.

6. Bonhoeffer, Dietrich, Life Together (New York: HarperCollins Publishers, 1954), 21.

7. Putnam, Robert D., *Bowling Alone* (New York: Simon and Schuster, 2000).

8. Marche, Stephen, *Is Facebook Making us Lonely?* The Atlantic, May, 2012.

9. Peck, M. Scott, *The Different Drum* (New York: Simon and Schuster, 1987), 86-106.

10. Zizza C., Siega-Riz AM, Popkin BM. *Significant increase in young adults' snacking between 1977-1978 and 1994-1996 represents a cause for concern!* Preventive Medicine 2001; 32:303. Bower, Del. "Cooking trends echo changing roles of women." Food Review 2000:23 (I):23-29. Cited from Food Politics, Nestle, Marion (Berkley and Los Angeles: University of California, 2002), 19.

11. Peck, M. Scott, *The Road Less Traveled* (New York: Simon and Schuster, 1978), 81.

12. Koenig, Harold, M.D., *The Healing Power of Faith* (Simon and Schuster, New York, 1999), 24.

13. Kolata, Gina, *Ultimate Fitness: The Quest for Truth about Exercise and Health* (New York: Farrar, Straus, and Giroux, 2003), 195.

14. Bartholomew, J., David Morrison, and Joseph Ciccolo. *"Effects of Acute Exercise on Mood and Well Being in Patients with Major Depressive Disorder,"* Medicine and Science in Sports and Exercise, Vol. 37, no. 12, Dec. 2005, 2032-37.

15. Covey, Stephen, *The 7 Habits of Highly Effective People* (New York: Simon and Schuster, 1989), 305.

16. Shaw, George Bernard (1856-1950), cited from Covey, 299.

17. Frankl, Viktor, *Man's Search for Meaning* (New York: Simon and Schuster, 1959), 48-49.

18.. Abner Hafer, my grandfather, died two months after the writing of this chapter at age ninety-four on August 18, 2005.

About the Author, Rev. Tom Hafer

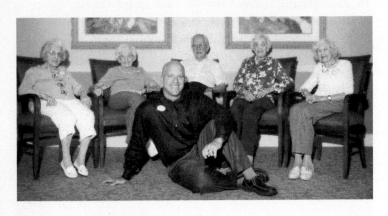

Author with five 100 year old residents of the community he serves as both Chaplain and Physical Therapist (gulfcoastvillage.com). They are living examples of the principles that are addressed in this book: healthy food, purposeful exercise, and a strong sense of community.
(photo-MelindaHawkins.com).

Books

Faith & Fitness: Diet and Exercise for a Better World
Revised and Updated
(Worzalla, 2012; 1st addition, Augsburg, 2007).

Aging Grace: The Journey to a Healthy 100
(Worzalla Publishing, 2012).

Wellplanet: Fitness as a Spiritual Discipline
(Worzalla Publishing, 2010).

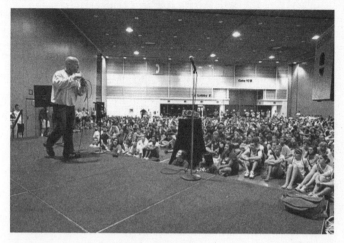

Tom Hafer has been lecturing throughout the country since 2002.
(photo: Faith & Fitness workshop, New Orleans, 2009).

Visit: **www.tomhafer.com**

and join the community that believes that our efforts made towards personal fitness can become a true spiritual discipline, an expression of gratitude, and thanksgiving for all of life. When we *care for ourselves to better care for others*, we simplify and intensify our quest for personal fitness.

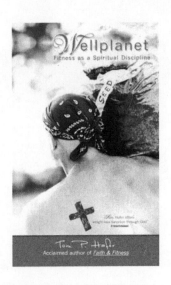

Wellplanet: Fitness as a Spiritual Discipline
Worzalla Publishing, 2010
(www.tomhafer.com)

Before becoming a monk, Brother Mark O'Reilly was an extraordinary small town physician. With his guru-like clarity, this 88 year old sage introduces Fitness as a Spiritual Discipline to his student, Hope. His timeless wisdom is for everyone who has fought the demons of weight-loss and won, then lost, then gained, then lost. For the sake of our personal health, our neighbor, and the planet; we have never had a timelier message to embrace...once again.

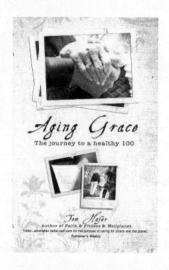

Aging Grace: The Journey to a Healthy 100

Worzalla Publishing, 2012

(www.tomhafer.com)

The Celtic Christians spoke of Thin Places 1500 years ago. These were said to be locations at which the separation between one's physical and spiritual worlds were paper thin. To live in a *Thin Place* is to be aware that our life is a journey. Although challenging at times, our lives are truly an orchestrated, harmonious God ordained pilgrimage; a long walk through Holy Ground. You will find that this spiritual discovery is a gift more precious than gold. In fact, besides *eating a healthy diet* and *having meaningful exercise* each day , this awareness could be thought of as the third variable that leads towards one-hundred years of healthy and inspired living. I invite you to discover your personal *Thin Place*, as you explore ours, at the Village.

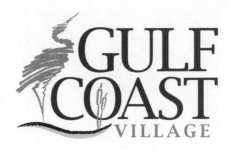

Gulf Coast Village is a Family of Senior Living Options that allows older Americans to maintain their independence and quality of life regardless of their current level of dependence. For twenty-five years, the focus of Gulf Coast Village Retirement Community has been to improve the quality of life for seniors in our community and provide the best health care possible. At the Village, we can provide everything from an occasional helping hand to full-time care. Our work touches the mind, body, heart — and ultimately the spirit — of those we served by integrating our deep compassion with highly effective programs and services for our residents, families, and the greater community we serve. *www.GulfCoastVillage.com*

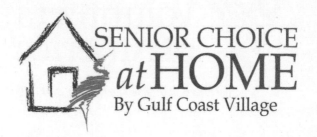

Senior Choice at Home by Gulf Coast Village is a unique membership–based program that offers comprehensive health care and personal assistance at home. This program is for older adults who must qualify while they are healthy and independent, offering financial security and peace of mind. If healthy senior living and being independent at home are important to you or a loved one, contact us today for more information. Geri Spaeth, *Executive Director of Senior Choice at Home. www.seniorchoiceathome.com*

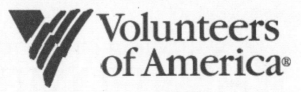

Volunteers of America®

There are no limits to caring.®

Volunteers of America is a national, nonprofit, faith-based organization dedicated to helping those in need live healthy, safe, and productive lives. Since 1896, our ministry of service has supported and empowered America's most vulnerable group, including: the frail elderly, people with disabilities, at-risk youth, men and women returning from prison, homeless individuals and families, those recovering from addictions, and many others. Through hundreds of human service programs including housing and health care; Volunteers of America helps more than 2 million people in over 400 communities. We offer a variety of services for older Americans, in particular, that allow them to maintain their independence and quality of life – everything from an occasional helping hand to full-time care. Our work touches the mind, body, heart — and ultimately the spirit — of those we serve by integrating our deep compassion with highly effective programs and services.

AGING WITH OPTIONS™

As one of the largest nonprofit providers of affordable senior housing in the United States, as well as a leading nonprofit provider of skilled nursing care and assisted living, Volunteers of America believes our mission today is to rise to the challenge of caring for an aging America.

With today's advancements in health care and special emphasis on preventive care; older Americans are experiencing a future of better health and longevity. No matter what stage of aging, no matter what state of health, Volunteers of America can offer the right support at the right time. We have the expertise to coordinate all the care and support necessary to meet each individual's needs, helping people maintain independence and self-sufficiency.

Building upon our long-established and trusted services for seniors, Aging with Options™ provides choices and support through each phase of life's journey. We do this through community engagement- home, community-based services, and the PACE (Program of All-inclusive Care for the Elderly) model of care management.

Volunteers of America invites everyone into its circle of caring and supports every older adult's right to age in place- surrounded by family and friends.